Hunger Satisfied Journal

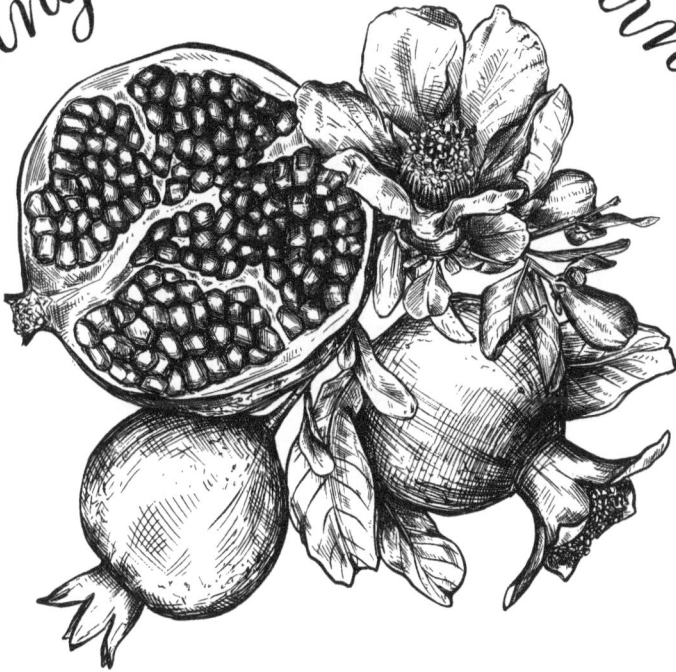

When you have eaten and are satisfied, you shall bless the LORD your God.

Deuteronomy 8:10

Annette Reeder

Designed Publishing, a division of Designed Healthy Living, Glen Allen, Virginia, 23059

Information contained in this journal is educational and merely offers nutritional support. It is not intended to replace medical advice. Seek a medical professional before making any changes to your diet or health program.

Unless otherwise noted, all Scriptures are taken from the Holy Bible, Scripture references marked kjv are taken from the King James Version of the Bible.

Scripture references marked nasb are taken from the New American Standard Bible, © 1960, 1963, 1968, 1971, 1972, 1973, 1975, 1977 by the Lockman Foundations. Used by permission.

Scripture references marked nkjv are taken from the New King James Version, © 1979, 1980, 1982 by Thomas Nelson, Inc., Publishers. Used by permission.

ISBN: 978-1-7376278-5-2 (paper back)
ISBN: 978-1-7376278-6-9 (Spiral bound)

dP
designed publishing

Welcome to a journal that will deliver the tools to a new understanding of God's love. God's love is expressed in multifaceted ways. The design of our bodies clearly demonstrates this love. Food was designed for nourishment and fellowship; this reveals a God who adores relationships. Our health also reveals His plan for us to prosper and be well when we follow biblical guidelines. Combine His foods with His design of our bodies, and His greatness becomes more evident.

Above all else may you prosper and be of good health. 3 John 3:2

Not only are we physical ~ We are spiritual
God works in our lives physically and spiritually!

This journal will connect the spiritual and the physical. The peace that is possible spiritually is also possible physically.

What if health was no longer an obstacle that kept you awake at night or in pain all the time or at a weight that was life altering?

What if food no longer plagued your mind but instead instilled it with peace and calmness?

Peace is possible, in who you are, what you eat, and your future health. And this journal is the best tool to see it happen.

God reveals Himself to each of us uniquely. Yet unhealthy and undisciplined eating can inhibit us from recognizing it. There is a mental and physical strain that accompanies undisciplined eating.

I am encouraged and enthused to share this valuable tool that has helped many people be set free to enjoy life abundantly. This tool will guide you to experience God's recipe for excellent health!

When you have eaten and are SATISFIED you shall bless the LORD your God for the good land which He has given you. Deuteronomy 8:10

Blessings to you as you discover Satisfied!

Annette Reeder

Tastimonies

Tastimony means letting your taste for God - His foods, His fellowship, and His plan to bring a change in your life that will flavor those around you, so they, too, desire the flavor of His grace.

For most of my life, and I'm almost 63, I have had numerous health issues. All praise goes to the Lord, that **most of these health issues have/are disappearing**. I basically am still eating mostly all plant-based foods, with salmon and eggs each a couple of times a week. This is the best I have felt for an exceedingly long time!! I thank and praise God, and thank you, Annette, for your wonderful ministry!! You are a wonderful blessing!! ~Diane W

I started this summer with the 40 Day Transformation and now it is early fall and I am **30 pounds lighter and no more meds!** My doctor said food did not matter. Now he is happy for me. I did exactly what Annette said, and I now look forward to meal time, knowing my body needs the nutrition and I am no longer eating for comfort. ~JP

I needed this years ago, yet here I am in my 40's and overweight. Through the 40 Day Transformation and this journal I have my life back! **I lost the weight and feel great!** Thanks. ~ S Davis

I learned to love fiber, and through this journal as a tool my cholesterol **dropped 30 points** in less than 30 days. I love the new foods – real foods. I can follow the 3 principles and know I will be healthy going forward. ~D Hughes

I played around with this tool and used it as a record of what I already ate. Then when I learned in the 40 Day Transformation coaching how to use it right – the **weight started dropping** quickly. This really works. And I hate journaling! ~S Heron

What to Expect

This Hunger ~ Satisfied Journal tracks progress and success. Some days will be hard, and other days will be incredibly joyful.

When a house is built, it seems the clearing of the land and the pouring of the footings are a slow process. No visible house. Yet the footings create a solid foundation that is stable during storms. The same is true of health. This journal sets the footings for a lifetime of success. It may seem slow at first, yet, believe me, the results will amaze you!

This journal can help these challenges:

- food sensitivities
- weight gain
- weight loss
- forgiveness
- health gain
- health maintanence
- exercise
- sleep

Plus, the mental shift learned from applying this journal will show you success for the rest of your life. Never again even say the word – *diet*!

Never say: *I need TO GET healthy.* You will be there and always know how to maintain it.

Your new phrase: *I am Satisfied!*

The results from using this journal *as instructed* – no wavering - will be:

- ♣ No longer challenged with food
- ♣ No longer binge/purge/overeating/mindless eating
- ♣ Feel amazing and in control
- ♣ Feel the true gift of health God promised
- ♣ Recognize and respond to the body's cues with satisfaction

Which one of these results excites you the most?

What if it could happen sooner with less effort?

How to Get Started

1. **Read all** of the instructions. This journal has been used in all coaching groups through The Biblical Nutrition Academy, and those who did not follow **all** the instructions did not see results as quickly. When they went back and read it thoroughly and joined the Inner Circle group, expectations were exceeded.

2. **Journal**; it has been proven those who journal have a 70% higher success rate over those who do not. This journal has several built-in steps to guarantee success happens quickly. Study each segment dutifully for the best start.

3. **Join** a coaching group. Accountability along with a coach is incredibly valuable. Jesus not only taught his disciples, but He coached them to help them visualize what they were thinking and whether their thoughts were in agreement with His Words. Go to https://thebiblicalnutritionist.com/biblical-health-inner-circle/ to sign up for the next coaching group. Working with our team of trained coaches makes this journey more enjoyable and more successful. Every coach has walked this journey before you and they know how to avoid the pitfalls and reach for the best results.

Hunger Satisfied

Recognizing true hunger and true satisfaction is the key to success for weight management and health.

God designed our bodies to let us know hunger and satisfaction through the use of hormones. These hormones work beautifully when we have a healthy microbiome, eat God designed foods, and have biblical wisdom. These signals are difficult to recognize when we consume addictive or processed foods, have a hormone imbalance, or have mental conditioning by advertisers, in addition to any personal misunderstanding of our own bodies.

Our goal with this journal is to help recognize hunger and learn to stop eating when satisfied. The more this happens, the sooner the hormones will balance and life will be grand.

We have an orchestrated group of hormones that signal when we are hungry, known as ghrelin, and when we are satisfied, known as leptin. Chemicals in our manipulated diet interfere with the communication, which silences true hunger or true fullness.

Good news!! God designed our bodies to heal.

Through the renewal in our cells and a rebuilding of the microbiome by eating God's foods, we can truly rebuild this system and become the naturally fit person God designed. To make this renewal happen, we need to focus on how we feel physically.

A healthy relationship with food is based on beliefs of who you are in Christ and the mutual desires of His design and your self-love to work together. With the right strategies everyone can gain the strength and courage needed to say "no more" to bad food.

When you know better, you do better. When you believe the Truth of God's Word, your health will reflect it.

Real knowledge of real food that builds healthy cells is the knowledge that builds a life of vigor.

Losing weight and feeling great is not about moderation or dieting; it is about developing good habits of eating the right foods and in the right amounts. It's about building and continually practicing good habits, not just in the area of your weight, but in all areas of your life.

People who manage stress, get enough sleep, and enjoy healthy, loving relationships have an easier time losing weight and keeping it off.

Hunger Signal

True hunger starts in the gut, not the mind. It is a growling or sensation that won't stop for minutes. It typically happens when there has been at least 4 hours since the last meal. Mental hunger is when you walk through the mall or grocery store and the aroma of cinnamon rolls is being wafted through the store. Just the smell makes you think "I want that!" but your body is not hungry.

Eating when we are not hungry is more likely to become stored energy and less likely to be utilized and burned. Stored energy can become fat. So eating when you are not hungry encourages your body to convert those unnecessary calories into fat.

YET, if you bypass that mental hunger and wait, your body will continue to BURN fat! Imagine the next time you want to eat while you are not truly hungry, Just say to yourself (or out loud), "Burn Baby Burn! Burn that FAT!"

If inflammation is a concern, then please note that fat contributes to inflammation. Reduce the fat in your body, and inflammation will be reduced.

Eating only when hungry allows the microbiome to reestablish a healthy microbiome. Continually grazing on food leads to an unhealthy microbiome. All health begins with a healthy microbiome. Even if weight loss is not your goal, eating ONLY when hungry is a dicipline that will transfer to other areas of your life.

Learn to Recognize Hunger

It is very likely that hunger signals are foreign to you. Here are some steps to learn the signals.

The first day of this journal plan to eat only half of a normal day's supply of food. This means eat a half breakfast such as 1 egg instead of 2 or ½ of a smoothie instead of a full smoothie. Then wait 4 hours untill lunch.

At lunch eat ½ sandwich and fruit. Then wait at least 4 hours till dinner and eat ½ your normal serving. By the next morning, hunger will likely be heard or felt. With the influx of chemicals in our diet, this may take 2-3 days of half eating to finally feel the true hunger sensation.

PLEASE DO NOT SKIP THIS STEP. THE SOONER HUNGER IS LEARNED THE MORE RAPID THE JOURNEY TO YOUR HEALTH SUCCESS!

Other Symptoms of Hunger or Poor Eating

Some people experience headaches or stomach pains when they are hungry or experience a glucose drop. As we implement a healthy diet this will disappear. If you do experience a headache and it is not attributed to sugar or caffeine withdrawal, drinking a 16-ounces glass of water may send it away. If the headache is a glucose drop headache, then add one organic apple. The headaches may happen less as your body starts to adapt to the healthy eating and timing of meals. This is also a symptom that change is very necessary to allow the body to better adapt to the use of glucose. Then try to wait untill the scheduled mealtime for the full meal.

The body is an incredible design. As you learn the signals you will be amazed at how it quickly adapts to a healthy diet. You may even enjoy eating kale ☺!

Satisfied Signal

Of the two signals, this is the most difficult. Were you told to "clean your plate", or "there are starving children in China, so eat everything!"? Does either of these make any sense? Yet, most of us have heard these or similar words. Are you still hungry even when you know you have eaten plenty? Do you finish a meal and then start grazing an hour later, looking for something salty or sweet?

These are all symptoms of addictions, hormonal imbalance, emotional instability, microbiome issues, and not understanding satisfied. Physically **satisfied**, or satiety, is a signal from the hormone leptin.

Eating continually and keeping blood glucose levels elevated can create leptin resistance. This leads to an almost impossible recognition of satiety.

This is fixable!

The "fix" is simple: it starts with eating God-designed foods, eating only when hungry, eating with four hours between meals, measuring out meals for healthy portions, and then sticking to that plan.

After a time of healing and no longer keeping an elevated blood glucose level, the leptin resistance will be lessened and satiety will be noticed.

Satiety is another word for **satisfied**.

Eating God's foods sets our hormones in balance once the microbiome is in balance. These hormones include the two we mentioned before: leptin and ghrelin. When these hormones are singing a happy tune, your level of satisfied in the body will bring you to a state of happiness that you will sing along! This includes signaling for **satisfied**.

Until we are completely reliant on our hormones to work, the use of this journal and the help of the coaching group are exceptional ways to learn how to train our thoughts for success.

To Learn "Satisfied":

- ♣ Stop halfway through a meal and pause.

- ♣ How do you feel at the halfway point?

- ♣ When the food stops tasting super good, you are satisfied.

- ♣ Eat slower. Allow your mind to catch up with your stomach.

- ♣ Set down your utensils between bites. Enjoy the food, bless the person who made it, praise God for His provisions, and ask for the recipe. These are all ways to be more mindful of the meal.

- ♣ The more we pause and praise, the easier and sooner it will be to recognize **satisfied**.

Satisfied Is Not:

- ✓ Unbuttoning your top button on your jeans.

- ✓ Eating till you are sick and want to vomit.

- ✓ Eating beyond a healthy portion.

- ✓ Craving food all day long.

What to Eat

3 Principles

1. Eat the foods God called GOOD for us to eat.

2. Eat the foods as close to His design as possible, before altering it beyond our health benefit.

3. Do not let any food become your god. Avoid addictions.

These principles helped me lose 60 pounds in the beginning of my journey. Now I use this journal to reach my goal, the most ideal weight and health.

To learn more about these principles read my book: *Treasures of Healthy Living Bible Study. thebiblicalnutritionist.com/Treasures*

Hunger – Satisfied Scale The KEY TO IT ALL!

Now let's make this journal work. Health starts by eating God designed foods and avoiding man's manipulated imitations.

Step one is knowing when to eat and when to stop. This is the step most coaches and diet books ignore. Because not only did God give us delicious foods that will bring health, but He built in signals that help us physically know when to eat and when to say, "I am Satisfied!"

Start each meal or snack by recording your hunger score. Then finish each eating time with a satisfied score.

In this journal we use one scale 1-10 to record both "Hunger" and "Satisfied."

Each scale should have two circles – the number you started the eating time and the number you stopped eating.

Example: Hunger /Fullness Scale: Starving 1 2③4 5 6 7 8⑨10 Stuffed

Here are some prompts to help:

On a scale of 1 – 10

1. Famished – I could eat the wallpaper, stomach growling

2. Hungry and ready to eat

3. I would like to eat very soon

4. Sort of hungry – getting ready

5. Neither hungry or satisfied

6. Starting to feel satisfied. Could stop and be fine. Stopping here would make you feel 'light'! A great feeling!

7. Comfortable – food no longer tastes amazing

8. Satisfied and feeling full – now is a good time to stop.

9. Too full – past satisfied – why am I still lifting my fork to my mouth?

10. Thanksgiving stuffed – gluttony – I don't like how I feel.

Ideally each meal time starts with a feeling of 2 and ends at a 6 or 7.

When you do this, give yourself credit!!! How did it feel?

If you miss the 7 mark, ask yourself "Why?" How did it feel? Was it worth it?

These questions will end the need for yo-yo dieting and forever dealing with health challenges.

The amazing feeling of satisfied begins when you are ready to be truly set free from health challenges within your control and living at the weight God designed for you. This feeling of SATISFIED is a new love for those who experience it!

> *When you have eaten and are SATISFIED you shall bless the*
> *LORD your God for the good land which He has given you.*
> *Deuteronomy 8:10*

REMEMBER:

Just as we are physical we are spiritual!

Just as we are spiritual we are physical!

Eating Satisfied

We were created to crave! Lysa TurKeurst wrote a New York Times bestseller: *Made To Crave* explaining this. Learning to eat only untill satisfied means we are willing to see what else we are craving. Food will never satisfy what God has intended for Himself. Food must never be our god. When we eat beyond satisfied we are elevating food above what God has planned and stepping away from His design.

Don't miss out! Learn the signals to enjoy **satisfied** and God's presence even more!

How To Use This Journal

1. **Start your day the Amen way.** The first thoughts of the day shape our day. As I teach in videos and conferences, when we wake up, the best way to make sure we are focused on seeing God at work, it is say outloud as soon as our feet hit the floor: Today is going to be an Amen Day! I heartily agree with what God brings my way. Now our day is ready for excelling still more.

2. **Plan your meals 24 hours in advance.** This is particularly important. Through this step we learn not to 'cheat' or rethink our plan. If changes need to be made, they are made the next day. What you write on Sunday for Monday is what you eat on Monday. No changes allowed. If you find yourself too hungry on Monday, adjust it for Tuesday. If you find yourself too full, then stop when you feel satisfied. Do not eat beyond satisfied. (More on this next.)

3. **Learn the Hunger Satisfied Cues** (signals). Record your scale at each meal. **See instructions in prior section.**

4. **Credits.** Every day give yourself minimum 3 credits for doing well. This can be credits for any area of your life including eating. Our focus is to be on what we did well and not where we messed up. Never serve guilt with a meal.

   Our culture says – you ate that cake, so the day is shot. What we are changing is looking at what we did right and focusing on that. The more we focus on what we did correctly, the more consistent our success will be and the more we can share in God's love.

   His love is everlasting, yet when we focus on our failures, we take on the belief that God does not love us. This is not true!

   Pride is focusing on our failures. Humbleness is focusing on the good in our life and praising God for it.

   Write these credits in the journal daily.

   Examples of credits:

   - I fasted 12 hours today – Yippee!

   - I walked 20 minutes today – super

   - I ate lots of fiber today!

   - I woke up and said *Today is going to be an Amen day*!

   - I followed my 24-hour plan completely!

5. **Advantage.** Write one advantage for following a healthy eating plan. This can be the same for several days or it can be different.

   Examples of Advantages:

   - I will feel amazing and energized playing with my kids or grandkids

   - I will look better

   - My breathing will be easier

   - I will sleep great

   - I will have no more pain

   - I will honor God with my body

6. **Bible Verse** – Read the Bible verse at the beginning of each day.

7. **Supplements** – a healthy body needs to supplement. The most necessary are multi vitamins, probiotic, vitamin D, magnesium, and Omega. Track your daily intake of supplements.

8. **Water.** Track your intake of water. Try to take in 16 ounces of water when you first awake daily. Each number on the journal represents 1 glass of 8 ounces.

9. **Record all food consumed.** Hopefully all meals are planned before bedtime the day defore. If you eat beyond what was planned or ate something not planned, write

down all food consumed. This will help you learn any food triggers or emotional triggers.

10. **Answer the questions**. At the end of each day answer the questions. These can also become credits. Congratulate yourself for every YES!

11. **Journal**. Use the journal space to write how you feel, a prayer to God, why you ate, and plans for the future. **Please do not pass this up.** As you write notes in this journal it will continue to reveal what is working and what is not.

    Journal how you feel after eating specific foods. This will help reveal food sensitivities. A food sensitivity can be revealed by how you feel from 2 to 72 hours after a meal. This journal will help you discover these sensitivities and then plan alternatives.

    If you ate a food not planned, how did you feel afterward? Were you sick or not mentally sharp? Write about it!

    The more you write the more will be revealed about your health and how you can see problems and make changes.

The value of this journal is only limited by your willingness to journal.

The more you journal the more change happens!! Be honest! Breakthroughs are coming!

My Advantage
*To be healthy
so I don't
have to 'get
healthy!*

*Today was a
little hard,
but when I
realized my
appetite and
hunger can
be controlled
and I will
see results -
it was worth
a little
anxiousness.*

Day ___: Make Today an Amen Day

*Whatever you do in word or deed, do all in the
name of the Lord Jesus, giving thanks through
Him to God the Father.*

Colossians 3:17

Date _____   Water 1 2 3 4 5 6 7 8 9

Breakfast   Time 8 am _____
                                        (fast 14 hours
Hunger/Fullness Scale:
Starving 1 (2) 3 4 5 6 7 (8) 9 10 Stuffed
Foods/Amounts
*2/3 cup Greek yogurt, 1 scoop protein, 5 pecan
halves, ½ apple, ¼ cup almond milk*

Lunch   Time 12:30 pm _____
                                        (fast 4-1/2 hours)
Hunger/Fullness Scale:
Starving 1 2 (3) 4 5 6 7 (8) 9 10 Stuffed
Foods/Amounts
*4 ounces tuna, with half avocado, on lettuce and
a grapefruit*

Dinner   Time 5:30 pm _____
Hunger/Fullness Scale:
Starving 1 (2) 3 4 5 6 7 (8) 9 10 Stuffed
Foods/Amounts
*Roasted chicken, roasted apples, butternut squash,
salad with cucumbers, tomatoes, and balsamic
vinegar for dressing. Largest organic apple I can
find for dessert*

🥨 *Snack*   Time _____

Hunger/Fullness Scale:

Starving 1 2 3 4 5 6 7 8 9 10 Stuffed

Foods/Amounts

no snacks planned today

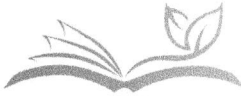

Journal

Was the food planned prior to starting the day?

☒ Yes   ❏ No

How many days have you followed a plan? _____

This is my first day toenjoy control! I can do it again!

Did you follow your plan?

☒ Yes   ❏ No

If not, why? If yes – how did it feel?

3 Credits

I followed my plan!!!

I started with an Amen Day - I can do that again!

I went outside when I thought of food and it was not time to eat!

Vitamins:

Multi • Probiotic • B Complex • Vitamin D
Calcium/Magnesium • Omega

What is Your Vision of the New You?

The heart of man plans his way,
but the Lord establishes his steps.
—Proverbs 16:9

The vision is important because it gives your life/health journey direction. Your vision is a combination of your dreams, your ideas about the life you want to live and your vision of what can happen in the next 60 days.

Challenge yourself to not only dream big but to dream better.

Use this page as a checklist of accomplishments. Refer back to this as your physical and spiritual goals keep increasing.

In the 40 Day Transformation course you were asked to write out your beliefs. This page here can be used to write them out and keep them close as you are inspired through this journal and see God at work.

Commit your work to the Lord,
and your plans will be established.
—Proverbs 16:3

My vision for 60 days from today.

My vision for 7 days from today.

My vision for 21 days from today.

I am so excited to see this happen……..

What if it could happen sooner with less effort? It CAN!

May he grant you your heart's desire
and fulfill all your plans!
—Psalms 20:4

Weekly Reflection

Take 5 to 10 minutes to reflect on your week. Always start from the perspective of what went well. Glance back at your credits. Focusing on the accomplishments directs the brain to continue in that pattern. The pattern of success.

Anticipate what the next seven days may include. Reflect on your eating, beliefs, and transformation tools; what needs more focus? Continue to offer up your prayers with thanksgiving!

God is at work and this journal is tracking His unique character in YOUR life.

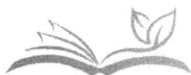

Prepare for the Next Week

As you review your personal calendar and see events or special gatherings, are there going to be any opportunities that may be a challenge?

Write that out now and decide how you are going to handle it.

Also make note of what days you are going to fast a meal. In the 40 Day Transformation Course it is taught for healthy living to fast 3 meals per week. These meals are totally your choice. Any day any meal.

Plan now your success in this area.

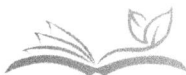

Day ___: Make Today an Amen Day

Whatever you do in word or deed, do all in the name of the Lord Jesus, giving thanks through Him to God the Father.

Colossians 3:17

Date _____   Water 1 2 3 4 5 6 7 8 9

Breakfast   Time _____
Hunger/Fullness Scale:

Starving   1   2   3   4   5   6   7   8   9   10   Stuffed
Foods/Amounts

Lunch   Time _____
Hunger/Fullness Scale:

Starving   1   2   3   4   5   6   7   8   9   10   Stuffed
Foods/Amounts

Dinner   Time _____
Hunger/Fullness Scale:

Starving   1   2   3   4   5   6   7   8   9   10   Stuffed
Foods/Amounts

🫐 *Snack*   Time _____

Hunger/Fullness Scale:

Starving   1   2   3   4   5   6   7   8   9   10   Stuffed

Foods/Amounts

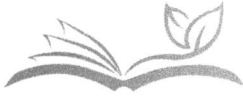

Was the food planned prior to starting the day?

❏ Yes   ❏ No

How many days have you followed a plan? _____

Did you follow your plan?

❏ Yes   ❏ No

If not, why? If yes – how did it feel?

Vitamins:

Multi • Probiotic • B Complex • Vitamin D
Calcium/Magnesium • Omega

Journal

3 Credits

Day ___: Make Today an Amen Day

Seek the Lord and His strength,
Seek His face continually.

1 Chronicles 16:11

Date _____   Water 1 2 3 4 5 6 7 8 9

🌿 *Breakfast*   Time _____
Hunger/Fullness Scale:
Starving 1 2 3 4 5 6 7 8 9 10 Stuffed
Foods/Amounts

🌿 *Lunch*   Time _____
Hunger/Fullness Scale:
Starving 1 2 3 4 5 6 7 8 9 10 Stuffed
Foods/Amounts

🌿 *Dinner*   Time _____
Hunger/Fullness Scale:
Starving 1 2 3 4 5 6 7 8 9 10 Stuffed
Foods/Amounts

🍩 *Snack* Time _____

Hunger/Fullness Scale:

Starving 1 2 3 4 5 6 7 8 9 10 Stuffed

Foods/Amounts

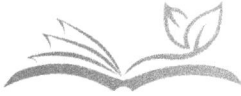

Was the food planned prior to starting the day?

❏ Yes ❏ No

How many days have you followed a plan? _____

Did you follow your plan?

❏ Yes ❏ No

If not, why? If yes – how did it feel?

Vitamins:

Multi • Probiotic • B Complex • Vitamin D
Calcium/Magnesium • Omega

My Advantage

Day ___: Make Today an Amen Day

*I have told you this so that my joy may be in
you and that your joy may be complete.*

John 15:11

Date _____   Water 1 2 3 4 5 6 7 8 9

🌿 *Breakfast*   Time _____
Hunger/Fullness Scale:

Starving   1   2   3   4   5   6   7   8   9   10   Stuffed

Foods/Amounts

🌿 *Lunch*   Time _____
Hunger/Fullness Scale:

Starving   1   2   3   4   5   6   7   8   9   10   Stuffed

Foods/Amounts

🌿 *Dinner*   Time _____
Hunger/Fullness Scale:

Starving   1   2   3   4   5   6   7   8   9   10   Stuffed

Foods/Amounts

🍳 *Snack*   Time _____

Hunger/Fullness Scale:

Starving   1   2   3   4   5   6   7   8   9   10   Stuffed

Foods/Amounts

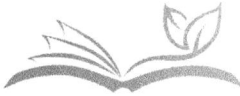

Was the food planned prior to starting the day?

❑ Yes   ❑ No

How many days have you followed a plan? _____

Did you follow your plan?

❑ Yes   ❑ No

If not, why? If yes – how did it feel?

Vitamins:

Multi • Probiotic • B Complex • Vitamin D
Calcium/Magnesium • Omega

Journal

3 Credits

My Advantage

Day ___: Make Today an Amen Day

So, whether you eat or drink or whatever you do,
do it all for the glory of God.

1 Corinthians 10:31

Date _____   Water 1 2 3 4 5 6 7 8 9

Breakfast   Time _____
Hunger/Fullness Scale:
Starving 1 2 3 4 5 6 7 8 9 10 Stuffed
Foods/Amounts

Lunch   Time _____
Hunger/Fullness Scale:
Starving 1 2 3 4 5 6 7 8 9 10 Stuffed
Foods/Amounts

Dinner   Time _____
Hunger/Fullness Scale:
Starving 1 2 3 4 5 6 7 8 9 10 Stuffed
Foods/Amounts

🫐 *Snack*   Time _____

Hunger/Fullness Scale:

Starving   1   2   3   4   5   6   7   8   9   10   Stuffed

Foods/Amounts

Journal

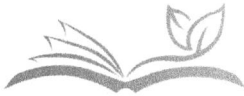

Was the food planned prior to starting the day?

❏ Yes   ❏ No

3 Credits

How many days have you followed a plan? _____

Did you follow your plan?

❏ Yes   ❏ No

If not, why? If yes – how did it feel?

Vitamins:

Multi • Probiotic • B Complex • Vitamin D
Calcium/Magnesium • Omega

My Advantage

Day ___: Make Today an Amen Day

Do not be conformed to this world, but be transformed by the renewing of your mind, so that you may prove what the will of God is, that which is good and acceptable and perfect.

Romans 12:2

Date _____   Water 1 2 3 4 5 6 7 8 9

Breakfast   Time _____
Hunger/Fullness Scale:
Starving 1 2 3 4 5 6 7 8 9 10 Stuffed
Foods/Amounts

Lunch   Time _____
Hunger/Fullness Scale:
Starving 1 2 3 4 5 6 7 8 9 10 Stuffed
Foods/Amounts

Dinner   Time _____
Hunger/Fullness Scale:
Starving 1 2 3 4 5 6 7 8 9 10 Stuffed
Foods/Amounts

🍩 *Snack*   Time _____

Hunger/Fullness Scale:

Starving 1 2 3 4 5 6 7 8 9 10 Stuffed

Foods/Amounts

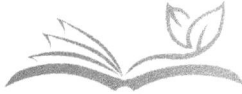

Was the food planned prior to starting the day?

❏ Yes   ❏ No

How many days have you followed a plan? _____

Did you follow your plan?

❏ Yes   ❏ No

If not, why? If yes – how did it feel?

Vitamins:

Multi • Probiotic • B Complex • Vitamin D
Calcium/Magnesium • Omega

Journal

3 Credits

Day ___: Make Today an Amen Day

*Therefore, I urge you, brothers and sisters,
in view of God's mercy, to offer your bodies
as a living sacrifice, holy and pleasing to God –
this is your true and proper worship.*

Romans 12:1

Date _____   Water 1 2 3 4 5 6 7 8 9

Breakfast   Time _____
Hunger/Fullness Scale:
Starving 1 2 3 4 5 6 7 8 9 10 Stuffed
Foods/Amounts

Lunch   Time _____
Hunger/Fullness Scale:
Starving 1 2 3 4 5 6 7 8 9 10 Stuffed
Foods/Amounts

Dinner   Time _____
Hunger/Fullness Scale:
Starving 1 2 3 4 5 6 7 8 9 10 Stuffed
Foods/Amounts

🍋 *Snack*　　　　Time _____

Hunger/Fullness Scale:

Starving　1　2　3　4　5　6　7　8　9　10　Stuffed

Foods/Amounts

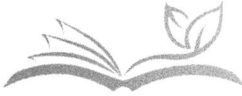

Was the food planned prior to starting the day?

❏ Yes　　❏ No

3 Credits

How many days have you followed a plan? _____

Did you follow your plan?

❏ Yes　　❏ No

If not, why? If yes – how did it feel?

Vitamins:

Multi • Probiotic • B Complex • Vitamin D
Calcium/Magnesium • Omega

My Advantage

Day ___: Make Today an Amen Day

You did not choose me, but I chose you and appointed you so that you might go and bear fruit – fruit that will last and so that whatever you ask in my name the Father will give you.

John 15:16

Date _____   Water 1 2 3 4 5 6 7 8 9

Breakfast   Time _____
Hunger/Fullness Scale:
Starving 1 2 3 4 5 6 7 8 9 10 Stuffed
Foods/Amounts

Lunch   Time _____
Hunger/Fullness Scale:
Starving 1 2 3 4 5 6 7 8 9 10 Stuffed
Foods/Amounts

Dinner   Time _____
Hunger/Fullness Scale:
Starving 1 2 3 4 5 6 7 8 9 10 Stuffed
Foods/Amounts

🫓 *Snack*   Time _____

Hunger/Fullness Scale:

Starving   1   2   3   4   5   6   7   8   9   10   Stuffed

Foods/Amounts

Journal

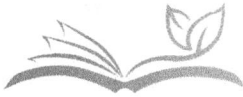

Was the food planned prior to starting the day?

❑ Yes   ❑ No

3 Credits

How many days have you followed a plan? _____

Did you follow your plan?

❑ Yes   ❑ No

If not, why? If yes – how did it feel?

Vitamins:

Multi • Probiotic • B Complex • Vitamin D
Calcium/Magnesium • Omega

Weekly Reflection

Take 5 to 10 minutes to reflect on your week. Always start from the perspective of what went well. Glance back at your credits. Focusing on the accomplishments directs the brain to continue in that pattern. The pattern of success.

Anticipate what the next seven days may include. Reflect on your eating, beliefs, and transformation tools; what needs more focus? Continue to offer up your prayers with thanksgiving!

God is at work and this journal is tracking His unique character in YOUR life.

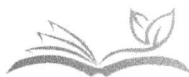

Prepare for the Next Week

As you review your personal calendar and see events or special gatherings, are there going to be any opportunities that may be a challenge?

Write that out now and decide how you are going to handle it.

Also make note of what days you are going to fast a meal. In the 40 Day Transformation Course it is taught for healthy living to fast 3 meals per week. These meals are totally your choice. Any day any meal.

Plan now your success in this area.

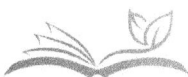

My Advantage

Day __: Make Today an Amen Day

Trust in the Lord with all your heart and
do not lean on your own understanding.
In all your ways acknowledge Him, and
He will make your paths straight.

Proverbs 3:5-6

Date _____   Water 1 2 3 4 5 6 7 8 9

Breakfast   Time _____
Hunger/Fullness Scale:
Starving   1   2   3   4   5   6   7   8   9   10   Stuffed
Foods/Amounts

Lunch   Time _____
Hunger/Fullness Scale:
Starving   1   2   3   4   5   6   7   8   9   10   Stuffed
Foods/Amounts

Dinner   Time _____
Hunger/Fullness Scale:
Starving   1   2   3   4   5   6   7   8   9   10   Stuffed
Foods/Amounts

🍩 *Snack*   Time _____

Hunger/Fullness Scale:

Starving 1 2 3 4 5 6 7 8 9 10 Stuffed

Foods/Amounts

Journal

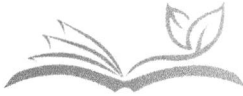

Was the food planned prior to starting the day?

❏ Yes   ❏ No

3 Credits

How many days have you followed a plan? _____

Did you follow your plan?

❏ Yes   ❏ No

If not, why? If yes – how did it feel?

Vitamins:

Multi • Probiotic • B Complex • Vitamin D
Calcium/Magnesium • Omega

Day ___: Make Today an Amen Day

*Do not be wise in your own eyes; fear the Lord
and turn away from evil. It will be healing
to your body and refreshment to your bones.*

Proverbs 3:7-8

Date _____   Water 1 2 3 4 5 6 7 8 9

Breakfast   Time _____
Hunger/Fullness Scale:
Starving 1 2 3 4 5 6 7 8 9 10 Stuffed
Foods/Amounts

Lunch   Time _____
Hunger/Fullness Scale:
Starving 1 2 3 4 5 6 7 8 9 10 Stuffed
Foods/Amounts

Dinner   Time _____
Hunger/Fullness Scale:
Starving 1 2 3 4 5 6 7 8 9 10 Stuffed
Foods/Amounts

🪷 *Snack*　　　　Time _____

Hunger/Fullness Scale:

Starving　1　2　3　4　5　6　7　8　9　10　Stuffed

Foods/Amounts

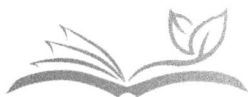

Was the food planned prior to starting the day?

❏ Yes　　❏ No

How many days have you followed a plan? _____

Did you follow your plan?

❏ Yes　　❏ No

If not, why? If yes – how did it feel?

Vitamins:

Multi • Probiotic • B Complex • Vitamin D
Calcium/Magnesium • Omega

Journal

3 Credits

Day ___: Make Today an Amen Day

If Your law had not been my delight, then I would have perished in my affliction. I will never forget Your precepts, for by them You have revived me.

Psalm 119:92-93

Date _____   Water 1 2 3 4 5 6 7 8 9

Breakfast   Time _____
Hunger/Fullness Scale:

Starving 1 2 3 4 5 6 7 8 9 10 Stuffed

Foods/Amounts

Lunch   Time _____
Hunger/Fullness Scale:

Starving 1 2 3 4 5 6 7 8 9 10 Stuffed

Foods/Amounts

Dinner   Time _____
Hunger/Fullness Scale:

Starving 1 2 3 4 5 6 7 8 9 10 Stuffed

Foods/Amounts

🍩 *Snack*   Time _____

Hunger/Fullness Scale:

Starving   1   2   3   4   5   6   7   8   9   10   Stuffed

Foods/Amounts

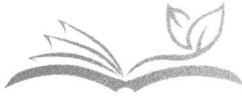

Was the food planned prior to starting the day?

❏ Yes   ❏ No

How many days have you followed a plan? _____

Did you follow your plan?

❏ Yes   ❏ No

If not, why? If yes – how did it feel?

Vitamins:

Multi • Probiotic • B Complex • Vitamin D
Calcium/Magnesium • Omega

3 Credits

Day ___: Make Today an Amen Day

The unfolding of Your words gives light;
it gives understanding to the simple.

Psalm 119:130

Date _____   Water 1 2 3 4 5 6 7 8 9

Breakfast   Time _____
Hunger/Fullness Scale:

Starving 1 2 3 4 5 6 7 8 9 10 Stuffed

Foods/Amounts

Lunch   Time _____
Hunger/Fullness Scale:

Starving 1 2 3 4 5 6 7 8 9 10 Stuffed

Foods/Amounts

Dinner   Time _____
Hunger/Fullness Scale:

Starving 1 2 3 4 5 6 7 8 9 10 Stuffed

Foods/Amounts

🍏 *Snack*   Time _____

Hunger/Fullness Scale:

Starving 1 2 3 4 5 6 7 8 9 10 Stuffed

Foods/Amounts

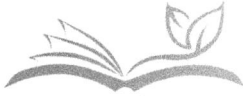

Was the food planned prior to starting the day?

❏ Yes   ❏ No

How many days have you followed a plan? _____

Did you follow your plan?

❏ Yes   ❏ No

If not, why? If yes – how did it feel?

Vitamins:

Multi • Probiotic • B Complex • Vitamin D
Calcium/Magnesium • Omega

Day ___: Make Today an Amen Day

My son, do not forget my teaching, but let your heart
keep my commandments; for length of days and
years of life and peace they will add to you.

Proverbs 3:1-2

Date _____   Water 1 2 3 4 5 6 7 8 9

Breakfast   Time _____
Hunger/Fullness Scale:
Starving 1   2   3   4   5   6   7   8   9   10   Stuffed
Foods/Amounts

Lunch   Time _____
Hunger/Fullness Scale:
Starving 1   2   3   4   5   6   7   8   9   10   Stuffed
Foods/Amounts

Dinner   Time _____
Hunger/Fullness Scale:
Starving 1   2   3   4   5   6   7   8   9   10   Stuffed
Foods/Amounts

🍪 *Snack*   Time _____

Hunger/Fullness Scale:

Starving   1   2   3   4   5   6   7   8   9   10   Stuffed

Foods/Amounts

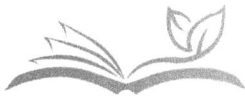

Was the food planned prior to starting the day?

❑ Yes   ❑ No

How many days have you followed a plan? _____

Did you follow your plan?

❑ Yes   ❑ No

If not, why? If yes – how did it feel?

Vitamins:

Multi • Probiotic • B Complex • Vitamin D
Calcium/Magnesium • Omega

Journal

My Advantage

Day ___: Make Today an Amen Day

And He has said to me, "My grace is sufficient for you, for power is perfected in weakness."

2 Corinthians 12:9

Date _____   Water 1 2 3 4 5 6 7 8 9

Breakfast   Time _____
Hunger/Fullness Scale:
Starving 1 2 3 4 5 6 7 8 9 10 Stuffed
Foods/Amounts

Lunch   Time _____
Hunger/Fullness Scale:
Starving 1 2 3 4 5 6 7 8 9 10 Stuffed
Foods/Amounts

Dinner   Time _____
Hunger/Fullness Scale:
Starving 1 2 3 4 5 6 7 8 9 10 Stuffed
Foods/Amounts

🥨 *Snack* Time _____

Hunger/Fullness Scale:

Starving 1 2 3 4 5 6 7 8 9 10 Stuffed

Foods/Amounts

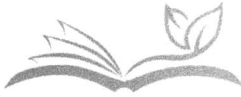

Was the food planned prior to starting the day?

❏ Yes   ❏ No

How many days have you followed a plan? _____

Did you follow your plan?

❏ Yes   ❏ No

If not, why? If yes – how did it feel?

Vitamins:

Multi • Probiotic • B Complex • Vitamin D

Calcium/Magnesium • Omega

Journal

3 Credits

Day ___: Make Today an Amen Day

The conclusion, when all has been heard, is:
fear God and keep His commandments,
because this applies to every person.

Ecclesiastes 12:13

Date _____   Water 1 2 3 4 5 6 7 8 9

Breakfast   Time _____
Hunger/Fullness Scale:
Starving 1 2 3 4 5 6 7 8 9 10 Stuffed
Foods/Amounts

Lunch   Time _____
Hunger/Fullness Scale:
Starving 1 2 3 4 5 6 7 8 9 10 Stuffed
Foods/Amounts

Dinner   Time _____
Hunger/Fullness Scale:
Starving 1 2 3 4 5 6 7 8 9 10 Stuffed
Foods/Amounts

🫐 *Snack*   Time _____

Hunger/Fullness Scale:

Starving 1 2 3 4 5 6 7 8 9 10 Stuffed

Foods/Amounts

.

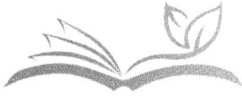

Was the food planned prior to starting the day?

❏ Yes   ❏ No

How many days have you followed a plan? _____

Did you follow your plan?

❏ Yes   ❏ No

If not, why? If yes – how did it feel?

Vitamins:

Multi • Probiotic • B Complex • Vitamin D
Calcium/Magnesium • Omega

Journal

3 Credits

Hunger ~ Satisfied Tastimony
Weekly Reflection

Take 5 to 10 minutes to reflect on your week. Always start from the perspective of what went well. Glance back at your credits. Focusing on the accomplishments directs the brain to continue in that pattern. The pattern of success.

Anticipate what the next seven days may include. Reflect on your eating, beliefs, and transformation tools; what needs more focus? Continue to offer up your prayers with thanksgiving!

God is at work and this journal is tracking His unique character in YOUR life.

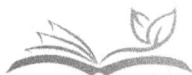

Prepare for the Next Week

As you review your personal calendar and see events or special gatherings, are there going to be any opportunities that may be a challenge?

Write that out now and decide how you are going to handle it.

Also make note of what days you are going to fast a meal. In the 40 Day Transformation Course it is taught for healthy living to fast 3 meals per week. These meals are totally your choice. Any day any meal.

Plan now your success in this area.

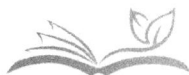

Day ___: Make Today an Amen Day

Therefore there is now no condemnation for those who are in Christ Jesus. For the law of the Spirit of life in Christ Jesus has set you free from the law of sin and of death.

Romans 8:1-2

Date _____   Water 1 2 3 4 5 6 7 8 9

🍳 Breakfast   Time _____
Hunger/Fullness Scale:

Starving 1 2 3 4 5 6 7 8 9 10 Stuffed

Foods/Amounts

🍳 Lunch   Time _____
Hunger/Fullness Scale:

Starving 1 2 3 4 5 6 7 8 9 10 Stuffed

Foods/Amounts

🍳 Dinner   Time _____
Hunger/Fullness Scale:

Starving 1 2 3 4 5 6 7 8 9 10 Stuffed

Foods/Amounts

🍩 *Snack*   Time _____

Hunger/Fullness Scale:

Starving 1 2 3 4 5 6 7 8 9 10 Stuffed

Foods/Amounts

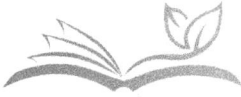

Was the food planned prior to starting the day?

❏ Yes   ❏ No

How many days have you followed a plan? _____

Did you follow your plan?

❏ Yes   ❏ No

If not, why? If yes – how did it feel?

Vitamins:

Multi • Probiotic • B Complex • Vitamin D

Calcium/Magnesium • Omega

Journal

3 Credits

My Advantage

Day ___: Make Today an Amen Day

For what the Law could not do, weak as it was
through the flesh, God did: sending His own Son
in the likeness of sinful flesh and as an offering
for sin, He condemned sin in the flesh.

Romans 8:3

Date _____   Water 1 2 3 4 5 6 7 8 9

Breakfast   Time _____
Hunger/Fullness Scale:
Starving   1   2   3   4   5   6   7   8   9   10   Stuffed
Foods/Amounts

Lunch   Time _____
Hunger/Fullness Scale:
Starving   1   2   3   4   5   6   7   8   9   10   Stuffed
Foods/Amounts

Dinner   Time _____
Hunger/Fullness Scale:
Starving   1   2   3   4   5   6   7   8   9   10   Stuffed
Foods/Amounts

🍪 *Snack*   Time _____

Hunger/Fullness Scale:

Starving 1 2 3 4 5 6 7 8 9 10 Stuffed

Foods/Amounts

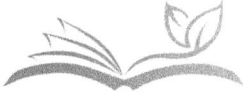

Was the food planned prior to starting the day?

❏ Yes   ❏ No

How many days have you followed a plan? _____

Did you follow your plan?

❏ Yes   ❏ No

If not, why? If yes – how did it feel?

Vitamins:

Multi • Probiotic • B Complex • Vitamin D
Calcium/Magnesium • Omega

My Advantage

Day ___: Make Today an Amen Day

There is a way which seems right to a man,
but its end is the way of death.

Proverbs 14:12

Date _____   Water 1 2 3 4 5 6 7 8 9

Breakfast   Time _____
Hunger/Fullness Scale:
Starving 1 2 3 4 5 6 7 8 9 10 Stuffed
Foods/Amounts

Lunch   Time _____
Hunger/Fullness Scale:
Starving 1 2 3 4 5 6 7 8 9 10 Stuffed
Foods/Amounts

Dinner   Time _____
Hunger/Fullness Scale:
Starving 1 2 3 4 5 6 7 8 9 10 Stuffed
Foods/Amounts

🍩 *Snack* Time _____

Hunger/Fullness Scale:

Starving 1 2 3 4 5 6 7 8 9 10 Stuffed

Foods/Amounts

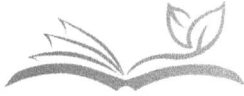

Was the food planned prior to starting the day?

❏ Yes   ❏ No

3 Credits

How many days have you followed a plan? _____

Did you follow your plan?

❏ Yes   ❏ No

If not, why? If yes – how did it feel?

Vitamins:

Multi • Probiotic • B Complex • Vitamin D
Calcium/Magnesium • Omega

Day ___: Make Today an Amen Day

You shall have no other gods before me.

Exodus 20:3

Date _____   Water 1 2 3 4 5 6 7 8 9

Breakfast   Time _____
Hunger/Fullness Scale:
Starving 1 2 3 4 5 6 7 8 9 10 Stuffed
Foods/Amounts

Lunch   Time _____
Hunger/Fullness Scale:
Starving 1 2 3 4 5 6 7 8 9 10 Stuffed
Foods/Amounts

Dinner   Time _____
Hunger/Fullness Scale:
Starving 1 2 3 4 5 6 7 8 9 10 Stuffed
Foods/Amounts

🍴 *Snack*　　　　Time _____

Hunger/Fullness Scale:

Starving　1　2　3　4　5　6　7　8　9　10　Stuffed

Foods/Amounts

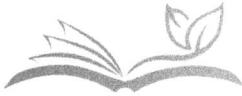

Was the food planned prior to starting the day?

❑ Yes　　❑ No

How many days have you followed a plan? _____

Did you follow your plan?

❑ Yes　　❑ No

If not, why? If yes – how did it feel?

Vitamins:

Multi • Probiotic • B Complex • Vitamin D
Calcium/Magnesium • Omega

Journal

3 Credits

Day ___: Make Today an Amen Day

*How blessed is the man who finds wisdom
and the man who gains understanding.*

Proverbs 3:13

Date _____   Water 1 2 3 4 5 6 7 8 9

Breakfast   Time _____
Hunger/Fullness Scale:

Starving 1 2 3 4 5 6 7 8 9 10 Stuffed

Foods/Amounts

Lunch   Time _____
Hunger/Fullness Scale:

Starving 1 2 3 4 5 6 7 8 9 10 Stuffed

Foods/Amounts

Dinner   Time _____
Hunger/Fullness Scale:

Starving 1 2 3 4 5 6 7 8 9 10 Stuffed

Foods/Amounts

🫐 *Snack* Time _____

Hunger/Fullness Scale:

Starving 1 2 3 4 5 6 7 8 9 10 Stuffed

Foods/Amounts

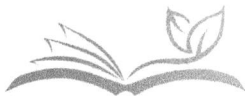

Was the food planned prior to starting the day?

❏ Yes   ❏ No

How many days have you followed a plan? _____

Did you follow your plan?

❏ Yes   ❏ No

If not, why? If yes – how did it feel?

Vitamins:

Multi • Probiotic • B Complex • Vitamin D
Calcium/Magnesium • Omega

Journal

3 Credits

Journal

My Advantage

Day ___: Make Today an Amen Day

The beginning of wisdom is: Acquire wisdom;
and with all your acquiring, get understanding.

Proverbs 4:7

Date _____   Water 1 2 3 4 5 6 7 8 9

Breakfast   Time _____
Hunger/Fullness Scale:
Starving   1   2   3   4   5   6   7   8   9   10   Stuffed
Foods/Amounts

Lunch   Time _____
Hunger/Fullness Scale:
Starving   1   2   3   4   5   6   7   8   9   10   Stuffed
Foods/Amounts

Dinner   Time _____
Hunger/Fullness Scale:
Starving   1   2   3   4   5   6   7   8   9   10   Stuffed
Foods/Amounts

🍽️ *Snack*　　　　　　　Time _____

Hunger/Fullness Scale:

Starving　1　2　3　4　5　6　7　8　9　10　Stuffed

Foods/Amounts

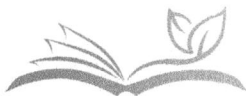

Was the food planned prior to starting the day?

❏ Yes　　❏ No

How many days have you followed a plan? _____

Did you follow your plan?

❏ Yes　　❏ No

If not, why? If yes – how did it feel?

Vitamins:

Multi • Probiotic • B Complex • Vitamin D
Calcium/Magnesium • Omega

Journal

3 Credits

Day ___: Make Today an Amen Day

*My son, give attention to my words; incline your
ear to my sayings. Do not let them depart from
your sight; keep them in the midst of your heart.*

Proverbs 4:20-22

Date _____   Water 1 2 3 4 5 6 7 8 9

Breakfast   Time _____
Hunger/Fullness Scale:

Starving 1 2 3 4 5 6 7 8 9 10 Stuffed

Foods/Amounts

Lunch   Time _____
Hunger/Fullness Scale:

Starving 1 2 3 4 5 6 7 8 9 10 Stuffed

Foods/Amounts

Dinner   Time _____
Hunger/Fullness Scale:

Starving 1 2 3 4 5 6 7 8 9 10 Stuffed

Foods/Amounts

🍩 *Snack*   Time _____

Hunger/Fullness Scale:

Starving   1   2   3   4   5   6   7   8   9   10   Stuffed

Foods/Amounts

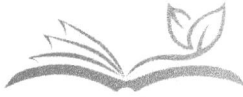

Was the food planned prior to starting the day?

❏ Yes   ❏ No

How many days have you followed a plan? _____

Did you follow your plan?

❏ Yes   ❏ No

If not, why? If yes – how did it feel?

Vitamins:

Multi • Probiotic • B Complex • Vitamin D
Calcium/Magnesium • Omega

3 Credits

Weekly Reflection

Take 5 to 10 minutes to reflect on your week. Always start from the perspective of what went well. Glance back at your credits. Focusing on the accomplishments directs the brain to continue in that pattern. The pattern of success.

Anticipate what the next seven days may include. Reflect on your eating, beliefs, and transformation tools; what needs more focus? Continue to offer up your prayers with thanksgiving!

God is at work and this journal is tracking His unique character in YOUR life.

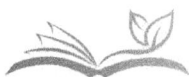

Prepare for the Next Week

As you review your personal calendar and see events or special gatherings, are there going to be any opportunities that may be a challenge?

Write that out now and decide how you are going to handle it.

Also make note of what days you are going to fast a meal. In the 40 Day Transformation Course it is taught for healthy living to fast 3 meals per week. These meals are totally your choice. Any day any meal.

Plan now your success in this area.

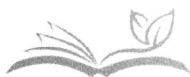

Day ___: Make Today an Amen Day

And the Lord will continually guide you, and satisfy your desire in scorched places, and give strength to your bones; and you will be like a watered garden, and like a spring of water whose waters do not fail.

Isaiah 58:11

Date _____   Water 1 2 3 4 5 6 7 8 9

Breakfast   Time _____
Hunger/Fullness Scale:
Starving 1 2 3 4 5 6 7 8 9 10 Stuffed
Foods/Amounts

Lunch   Time _____
Hunger/Fullness Scale:
Starving 1 2 3 4 5 6 7 8 9 10 Stuffed
Foods/Amounts

Dinner   Time _____
Hunger/Fullness Scale:
Starving 1 2 3 4 5 6 7 8 9 10 Stuffed
Foods/Amounts

🍽 *Snack* Time _____

Hunger/Fullness Scale:

Starving 1 2 3 4 5 6 7 8 9 10 Stuffed

Foods/Amounts

Journal

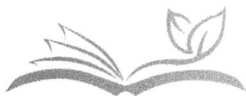

Was the food planned prior to starting the day?

❏ Yes   ❏ No

How many days have you followed a plan? _____

Did you follow your plan?

❏ Yes   ❏ No

If not, why? If yes – how did it feel?

Vitamins:

Multi • Probiotic • B Complex • Vitamin D
Calcium/Magnesium • Omega

3 Credits

Day ___: Make Today an Amen Day

The Lord will answer and say to His people, "Behold, I am going to send you grain, new wine and oil, and you will be satisfied in full with them; and I will never again make you a reproach among the nations."

Joel 2:19

Date _____   Water 1 2 3 4 5 6 7 8 9

Breakfast   Time _____
Hunger/Fullness Scale:
Starving   1   2   3   4   5   6   7   8   9   10   Stuffed
Foods/Amounts

Lunch   Time _____
Hunger/Fullness Scale:
Starving   1   2   3   4   5   6   7   8   9   10   Stuffed
Foods/Amounts

Dinner   Time _____
Hunger/Fullness Scale:
Starving   1   2   3   4   5   6   7   8   9   10   Stuffed
Foods/Amounts

🏌️ *Snack*   Time _____

Hunger/Fullness Scale:

Starving   1   2   3   4   5   6   7   8   9   10   Stuffed

Foods/Amounts

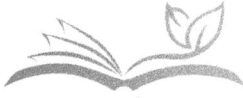

Was the food planned prior to starting the day?

❏ Yes   ❏ No

How many days have you followed a plan? _____

Did you follow your plan?

❏ Yes   ❏ No

If not, why? If yes – how did it feel?

Vitamins:

Multi • Probiotic • B Complex • Vitamin D
Calcium/Magnesium • Omega

Day ___: Make Today an Amen Day

...for you were formerly darkness, but now you are Light in the Lord; walk as children of Light (for the fruit of the Light consists in all goodness and righteousness and truth), trying to learn what is pleasing to the Lord.

Ephesians 5:8-10

Date _____   Water 1 2 3 4 5 6 7 8 9

Breakfast   Time _____
Hunger/Fullness Scale:
Starving 1 2 3 4 5 6 7 8 9 10 Stuffed
Foods/Amounts

Lunch   Time _____
Hunger/Fullness Scale:
Starving 1 2 3 4 5 6 7 8 9 10 Stuffed
Foods/Amounts

Dinner   Time _____
Hunger/Fullness Scale:
Starving 1 2 3 4 5 6 7 8 9 10 Stuffed
Foods/Amounts

🍪 *Snack* Time _____

Hunger/Fullness Scale:

Starving 1 2 3 4 5 6 7 8 9 10 Stuffed

Foods/Amounts

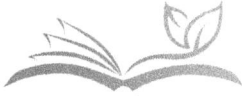

Was the food planned prior to starting the day?

❏ Yes   ❏ No

3 Credits

How many days have you followed a plan? _____

Did you follow your plan?

❏ Yes   ❏ No

If not, why? If yes – how did it feel?

Vitamins:

Multi • Probiotic • B Complex • Vitamin D
Calcium/Magnesium • Omega

Day ___: Make Today an Amen Day

Call to Me and I will answer you, and I will tell you
great and mighty things, which you do not know.
                                                    Jeremiah 33:3

Date _____   Water 1 2 3 4 5 6 7 8 9

Breakfast   Time _____
Hunger/Fullness Scale:
Starving 1 2 3 4 5 6 7 8 9 10 Stuffed
Foods/Amounts

Lunch   Time _____
Hunger/Fullness Scale:
Starving 1 2 3 4 5 6 7 8 9 10 Stuffed
Foods/Amounts

Dinner   Time _____
Hunger/Fullness Scale:
Starving 1 2 3 4 5 6 7 8 9 10 Stuffed
Foods/Amounts

🫐 *Snack*   Time _____

Hunger/Fullness Scale:

Starving   1   2   3   4   5   6   7   8   9   10   Stuffed

Foods/Amounts

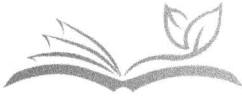

Was the food planned prior to starting the day?

❏ Yes   ❏ No

How many days have you followed a plan? _____

Did you follow your plan?

❏ Yes   ❏ No

If not, why? If yes – how did it feel?

Vitamins:

Multi • Probiotic • B Complex • Vitamin D
Calcium/Magnesium • Omega

Journal

3 Credits

My Advantage

Day ___: Make Today an Amen Day

He waters the mountains from His upper chambers; the earth is satisfied with the fruit of His works. He causes the grass to grow for the cattle, and vegetation for the labor of man, so that he may bring forth food from the earth.

Psalm 104:13-14

Date _____   Water 1 2 3 4 5 6 7 8 9

Breakfast   Time _____
Hunger/Fullness Scale:

Starving 1 2 3 4 5 6 7 8 9 10 Stuffed

Foods/Amounts

Lunch   Time _____
Hunger/Fullness Scale:

Starving 1 2 3 4 5 6 7 8 9 10 Stuffed

Foods/Amounts

Dinner   Time _____
Hunger/Fullness Scale:

Starving 1 2 3 4 5 6 7 8 9 10 Stuffed

Foods/Amounts

🍩 *Snack*   Time _____

Hunger/Fullness Scale:

Starving 1 2 3 4 5 6 7 8 9 10 Stuffed

Foods/Amounts

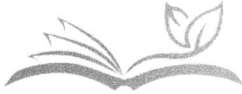

Was the food planned prior to starting the day?

❏ Yes   ❏ No

How many days have you followed a plan? _____

Did you follow your plan?

❏ Yes   ❏ No

If not, why? If yes – how did it feel?

Vitamins:

Multi • Probiotic • B Complex • Vitamin D
Calcium/Magnesium • Omega

Day ___: Make Today an Amen Day

He will be like a tree firmly planted by streams of water, which yields its fruit in its season and its leaf does not wither; and in whatever he does, he prospers.

Psalm 1:3

Date _____   Water 1 2 3 4 5 6 7 8 9

Breakfast   Time _____
Hunger/Fullness Scale:
Starving 1 2 3 4 5 6 7 8 9 10 Stuffed
Foods/Amounts

Lunch   Time _____
Hunger/Fullness Scale:
Starving 1 2 3 4 5 6 7 8 9 10 Stuffed
Foods/Amounts

Dinner   Time _____
Hunger/Fullness Scale:
Starving 1 2 3 4 5 6 7 8 9 10 Stuffed
Foods/Amounts

🥨 *Snack*　　　　　　Time _____

Hunger/Fullness Scale:

Starving　1　2　3　4　5　6　7　8　9　10　Stuffed

Foods/Amounts

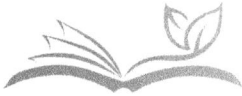

Was the food planned prior to starting the day?

❏ Yes　　❏ No

3 Credits

How many days have you followed a plan? _____

Did you follow your plan?

❏ Yes　　❏ No

If not, why? If yes – how did it feel?

Vitamins:

Multi • Probiotic • B Complex • Vitamin D

Calcium/Magnesium • Omega

Journal

My Advantage

Day ___: Make Today an Amen Day

The earth brought forth vegetation, plants yielding seed after their kind, and trees bearing fruit with seed in them, after their kind; and God saw that it was good.

Genesis 1:12

Date _____   Water 1 2 3 4 5 6 7 8 9

Breakfast   Time _____
Hunger/Fullness Scale:
Starving 1   2   3   4   5   6   7   8   9   10   Stuffed
Foods/Amounts

Lunch   Time _____
Hunger/Fullness Scale:
Starving 1   2   3   4   5   6   7   8   9   10   Stuffed
Foods/Amounts

Dinner   Time _____
Hunger/Fullness Scale:
Starving 1   2   3   4   5   6   7   8   9   10   Stuffed
Foods/Amounts

🥝 *Snack*   Time _____

Hunger/Fullness Scale:

Starving   1   2   3   4   5   6   7   8   9   10   Stuffed

Foods/Amounts

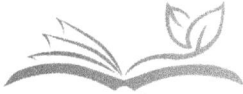

Was the food planned prior to starting the day?

❏ Yes   ❏ No

How many days have you followed a plan? _____

Did you follow your plan?

❏ Yes   ❏ No

If not, why? If yes – how did it feel?

Vitamins:

Multi • Probiotic • B Complex • Vitamin D
Calcium/Magnesium • Omega

Hunger ~ Satisfied Tastimony
Weekly Reflection

Take 5 to 10 minutes to reflect on your week. Always start from the perspective of what went well. Glance back at your credits. Focusing on the accomplishments directs the brain to continue in that pattern. The pattern of success.

Anticipate what the next seven days may include. Reflect on your eating, beliefs, and transformation tools; what needs more focus? Continue to offer up your prayers with thanksgiving!

God is at work and this journal is tracking His unique character in YOUR life.

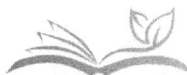

Prepare for the Next Week

As you review your personal calendar and see events or special gatherings, are there going to be any opportunities that may be a challenge?

Write that out now and decide how you are going to handle it.

Also make note of what days you are going to fast a meal. In the 40 Day Transformation Course it is taught for healthy living to fast 3 meals per week. These meals are totally your choice. Any day any meal.

Plan now your success in this area.

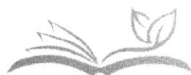

Day ___: Make Today an Amen Day

*There is an appointed time for everything.
And there is a time for every event under heaven—
a time to give birth and a time to die; a time to
plant and a time to uproot what is planted.*

Ecclesiastes 3:1-2

Date _____   Water 1 2 3 4 5 6 7 8 9

🌿 Breakfast   Time _____
Hunger/Fullness Scale:
Starving 1 2 3 4 5 6 7 8 9 10 Stuffed
Foods/Amounts

🌿 Lunch   Time _____
Hunger/Fullness Scale:
Starving 1 2 3 4 5 6 7 8 9 10 Stuffed
Foods/Amounts

🌿 Dinner   Time _____
Hunger/Fullness Scale:
Starving 1 2 3 4 5 6 7 8 9 10 Stuffed
Foods/Amounts

🍪 *Snack*   Time _____

Hunger/Fullness Scale:

Starving   1   2   3   4   5   6   7   8   9   10   Stuffed

Foods/Amounts

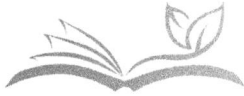

Was the food planned prior to starting the day?

❏ Yes   ❏ No

How many days have you followed a plan? _____

Did you follow your plan?

❏ Yes   ❏ No

If not, why? If yes – how did it feel?

Vitamins:

Multi • Probiotic • B Complex • Vitamin D
Calcium/Magnesium • Omega

Journal

3 Credits

Day ___: Make Today an Amen Day

And He said to them, "Because of the littleness of your faith;
for truly I say to you, if you have faith the size of a mustard
seed, you will say to this mountain, 'Move from here to there,'
and it will move; and nothing will be impossible to you."

Matthew 17:20

Date _____   Water 1 2 3 4 5 6 7 8 9

Breakfast   Time _____
Hunger/Fullness Scale:
Starving   1   2   3   4   5   6   7   8   9   10   Stuffed
Foods/Amounts

Lunch   Time _____
Hunger/Fullness Scale:
Starving   1   2   3   4   5   6   7   8   9   10   Stuffed
Foods/Amounts

Dinner   Time _____
Hunger/Fullness Scale:
Starving   1   2   3   4   5   6   7   8   9   10   Stuffed
Foods/Amounts

🥨 *Snack*   Time _____

Hunger/Fullness Scale:

Starving 1 2 3 4 5 6 7 8 9 10 Stuffed

Foods/Amounts

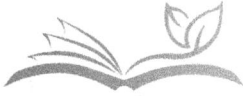

Was the food planned prior to starting the day?

❏ Yes   ❏ No

How many days have you followed a plan? _____

Did you follow your plan?

❏ Yes   ❏ No

If not, why? If yes – how did it feel?

Vitamins:

Multi • Probiotic • B Complex • Vitamin D
Calcium/Magnesium • Omega

Day ___: Make Today an Amen Day

Open my eyes, that I may behold
wonderful things from Your law.

Psalm 119:18

Date _____   Water 1 2 3 4 5 6 7 8 9

Breakfast   Time _____
Hunger/Fullness Scale:

Starving 1   2   3   4   5   6   7   8   9   10   Stuffed

Foods/Amounts

Lunch   Time _____
Hunger/Fullness Scale:

Starving 1   2   3   4   5   6   7   8   9   10   Stuffed

Foods/Amounts

Dinner   Time _____
Hunger/Fullness Scale:

Starving 1   2   3   4   5   6   7   8   9   10   Stuffed

Foods/Amounts

🍈 *Snack*   Time _____

Hunger/Fullness Scale:

Starving   1   2   3   4   5   6   7   8   9   10   Stuffed

Foods/Amounts

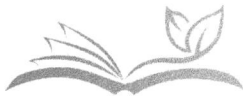

Was the food planned prior to starting the day?

❏ Yes   ❏ No

3 Credits

How many days have you followed a plan? _____

Did you follow your plan?

❏ Yes   ❏ No

If not, why? If yes – how did it feel?

Vitamins:

Multi • Probiotic • B Complex • Vitamin D
Calcium/Magnesium • Omega

Journal

My Advantage

Day ___: Make Today an Amen Day

Oh that they had such a heart in them, that they would fear Me and keep all My commandments always, that it may be well with them and with their sons forever!

Deuteronomy 5:29

Date _____   Water 1 2 3 4 5 6 7 8 9

Breakfast   Time _____
Hunger/Fullness Scale:
Starving 1 2 3 4 5 6 7 8 9 10 Stuffed
Foods/Amounts

Lunch   Time _____
Hunger/Fullness Scale:
Starving 1 2 3 4 5 6 7 8 9 10 Stuffed
Foods/Amounts

Dinner   Time _____
Hunger/Fullness Scale:
Starving 1 2 3 4 5 6 7 8 9 10 Stuffed
Foods/Amounts

🍪 *Snack*　　　　Time _____

Hunger/Fullness Scale:

Starving　1　2　3　4　5　6　7　8　9　10　Stuffed

Foods/Amounts

Journal

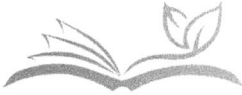

Was the food planned prior to starting the day?

❏ Yes　　❏ No

3 Credits

How many days have you followed a plan? _____

Did you follow your plan?

❏ Yes　　❏ No

If not, why? If yes – how did it feel?

Vitamins:

Multi • Probiotic • B Complex • Vitamin D
Calcium/Magnesium • Omega

Day ___: Make Today an Amen Day

For I am the Lord your God. Consecrate yourselves therefore, and be holy, for I am holy.

Leviticus 11:44a

Date _____   Water 1 2 3 4 5 6 7 8 9

Breakfast   Time _____
Hunger/Fullness Scale:

Starving 1 2 3 4 5 6 7 8 9 10 Stuffed

Foods/Amounts

Lunch   Time _____
Hunger/Fullness Scale:

Starving 1 2 3 4 5 6 7 8 9 10 Stuffed

Foods/Amounts

Dinner   Time _____
Hunger/Fullness Scale:

Starving 1 2 3 4 5 6 7 8 9 10 Stuffed

Foods/Amounts

🍪 *Snack*   Time _____

Hunger/Fullness Scale:

Starving 1 2 3 4 5 6 7 8 9 10 Stuffed

Foods/Amounts

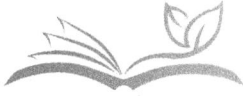

Was the food planned prior to starting the day?

❏ Yes   ❏ No

3 Credits

How many days have you followed a plan? _____

Did you follow your plan?

❏ Yes   ❏ No

If not, why? If yes – how did it feel?

Vitamins:

Multi • Probiotic • B Complex • Vitamin D
Calcium/Magnesium • Omega

Day ___: Make Today an Amen Day

*For everyone who asks, receives; and he who seeks, finds;
and to him who knocks, it will be opened.*

Luke 11:10

Date _____   Water 1 2 3 4 5 6 7 8 9

Breakfast   Time _____
Hunger/Fullness Scale:
Starving 1 2 3 4 5 6 7 8 9 10 Stuffed
Foods/Amounts

Lunch   Time _____
Hunger/Fullness Scale:
Starving 1 2 3 4 5 6 7 8 9 10 Stuffed
Foods/Amounts

Dinner   Time _____
Hunger/Fullness Scale:
Starving 1 2 3 4 5 6 7 8 9 10 Stuffed
Foods/Amounts

🫐 *Snack*   Time _____

Hunger/Fullness Scale:

Starving   1   2   3   4   5   6   7   8   9   10   Stuffed

Foods/Amounts

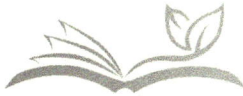

Was the food planned prior to starting the day?

❑ Yes   ❑ No

3 Credits

How many days have you followed a plan? _____

Did you follow your plan?

❑ Yes   ❑ No

If not, why? If yes – how did it feel?

Vitamins:

Multi • Probiotic • B Complex • Vitamin D
Calcium/Magnesium • Omega

Day ___: Make Today an Amen Day

Do not think that I came to abolish the Law or the Prophets; I did not come to abolish but to fulfill.

Matthew 5:17

Date _____   Water 1 2 3 4 5 6 7 8 9

Breakfast   Time _____

Hunger/Fullness Scale:

Starving 1 2 3 4 5 6 7 8 9 10 Stuffed

Foods/Amounts

Lunch   Time _____

Hunger/Fullness Scale:

Starving 1 2 3 4 5 6 7 8 9 10 Stuffed

Foods/Amounts

Dinner   Time _____

Hunger/Fullness Scale:

Starving 1 2 3 4 5 6 7 8 9 10 Stuffed

Foods/Amounts

Snack　　　　Time _____

Hunger/Fullness Scale:

Starving　1　2　3　4　5　6　7　8　9　10　Stuffed

Foods/Amounts

Journal

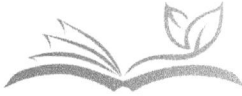

Was the food planned prior to starting the day?

❑ Yes　　❑ No

How many days have you followed a plan? _____

Did you follow your plan?

❑ Yes　　❑ No

If not, why? If yes – how did it feel?

Vitamins:

Multi • Probiotic • B Complex • Vitamin D
Calcium/Magnesium • Omega

3 Credits

Hunger ~ Satisfied Tastimony

Weekly Reflection

Take 5 to 10 minutes to reflect on your week. Always start from the perspective of what went well. Glance back at your credits. Focusing on the accomplishments directs the brain to continue in that pattern. The pattern of success.

Anticipate what the next seven days may include. Reflect on your eating, beliefs, and transformation tools; what needs more focus? Continue to offer up your prayers with thanksgiving!

God is at work and this journal is tracking His unique character in YOUR life.

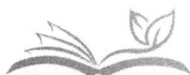

Prepare for the Next Week

As you review your personal calendar and see events or special gatherings, are there going to be any opportunities that may be a challenge?

Write that out now and decide how you are going to handle it.

Also make note of what days you are going to fast a meal. In the 40 Day Transformation Course it is taught for healthy living to fast 3 meals per week. These meals are totally your choice. Any day any meal.

Plan now your success in this area.

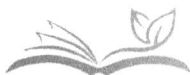

My Advantage

Day __: Make Today an Amen Day

*Discipline yourself for the purpose of godliness;
for bodily discipline is only of little profit, but godliness
is profitable for all things, since it holds promise for
the present life and also for the life to come.*

1 Timothy 4:7b-8

Date _____   Water 1 2 3 4 5 6 7 8 9

🥚 Breakfast   Time _____
Hunger/Fullness Scale:

Starving 1 2 3 4 5 6 7 8 9 10 Stuffed
Foods/Amounts

🥗 Lunch   Time _____
Hunger/Fullness Scale:

Starving 1 2 3 4 5 6 7 8 9 10 Stuffed
Foods/Amounts

🍽 Dinner   Time _____
Hunger/Fullness Scale:

Starving 1 2 3 4 5 6 7 8 9 10 Stuffed
Foods/Amounts

🥗 *Snack*   Time _____

Hunger/Fullness Scale:

Starving   1   2   3   4   5   6   7   8   9   10   Stuffed

Foods/Amounts

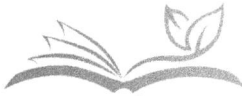

Was the food planned prior to starting the day?

❏ Yes   ❏ No

How many days have you followed a plan? _____

Did you follow your plan?

❏ Yes   ❏ No

If not, why? If yes – how did it feel?

Vitamins:

Multi • Probiotic • B Complex • Vitamin D
Calcium/Magnesium • Omega

Journal

3 Credits

Day ___: Make Today an Amen Day

*Do not be with heavy drinkers of wine,
or with gluttonous eaters of meat; for the heavy
drinker and the glutton will come to poverty,
and drowsiness will clothe one with rags.*

Proverbs 23:20-21

Date _____   Water 1 2 3 4 5 6 7 8 9

Breakfast   Time _____
Hunger/Fullness Scale:
Starving 1 2 3 4 5 6 7 8 9 10 Stuffed
Foods/Amounts

Lunch   Time _____
Hunger/Fullness Scale:
Starving 1 2 3 4 5 6 7 8 9 10 Stuffed
Foods/Amounts

Dinner   Time _____
Hunger/Fullness Scale:
Starving 1 2 3 4 5 6 7 8 9 10 Stuffed
Foods/Amounts

Snack   Time _____

Hunger/Fullness Scale:

Starving 1 2 3 4 5 6 7 8 9 10 Stuffed

Foods/Amounts

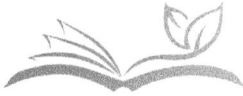

Was the food planned prior to starting the day?

❏ Yes   ❏ No

3 Credits

How many days have you followed a plan? _____

Did you follow your plan?

❏ Yes   ❏ No

If not, why? If yes – how did it feel?

Vitamins:

Multi • Probiotic • B Complex • Vitamin D
Calcium/Magnesium • Omega

Day ___: Make Today an Amen Day

*For I know the plans that I have for you,
declares the Lord, plans for welfare and not for
calamity to give you a future and a hope.*

Jeremiah 29:11

Date _____   Water 1 2 3 4 5 6 7 8 9

Breakfast   Time _____
Hunger/Fullness Scale:

Starving   1   2   3   4   5   6   7   8   9   10   Stuffed

Foods/Amounts

Lunch   Time _____
Hunger/Fullness Scale:

Starving   1   2   3   4   5   6   7   8   9   10   Stuffed

Foods/Amounts

Dinner   Time _____
Hunger/Fullness Scale:

Starving   1   2   3   4   5   6   7   8   9   10   Stuffed

Foods/Amounts

🫓 *Snack*　　　　　　Time _____

Hunger/Fullness Scale:

Starving 1 2 3 4 5 6 7 8 9 10 Stuffed

Foods/Amounts

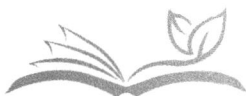

Was the food planned prior to starting the day?

❏ Yes　　❏ No

How many days have you followed a plan? _____

Did you follow your plan?

❏ Yes　　❏ No

If not, why? If yes – how did it feel?

Vitamins:

Multi • Probiotic • B Complex • Vitamin D
Calcium/Magnesium • Omega

Journal

3 Credits

Day ___: Make Today an Amen Day

Then you will call upon Me and come and pray to Me, and I will listen to you. You will seek Me and find Me when you search for Me with all your heart.

Jeremiah 29:12-13

Date _____   Water 1 2 3 4 5 6 7 8 9

🍴 *Breakfast*   Time _____
Hunger/Fullness Scale:

Starving 1   2   3   4   5   6   7   8   9   10   Stuffed

Foods/Amounts

🍴 *Lunch*   Time _____
Hunger/Fullness Scale:

Starving 1   2   3   4   5   6   7   8   9   10   Stuffed

Foods/Amounts

🍴 *Dinner*   Time _____
Hunger/Fullness Scale:

Starving 1   2   3   4   5   6   7   8   9   10   Stuffed

Foods/Amounts

🥐 *Snack* Time _____

Hunger/Fullness Scale:

Starving 1 2 3 4 5 6 7 8 9 10 Stuffed

Foods/Amounts

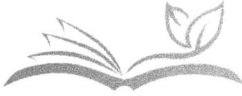

Was the food planned prior to starting the day?

❏ Yes   ❏ No

How many days have you followed a plan? _____

Did you follow your plan?

❏ Yes   ❏ No

If not, why? If yes – how did it feel?

Vitamins:

Multi • Probiotic • B Complex • Vitamin D
Calcium/Magnesium • Omega

Journal

3 Credits

My Advantage

Day ___: Make Today an Amen Day

For a righteous man falls seven times, and rises again,
but the wicked stumble in time of calamity.

Proverbs 24:16

Date _____   Water 1 2 3 4 5 6 7 8 9

Breakfast   Time _____
Hunger/Fullness Scale:
Starving   1   2   3   4   5   6   7   8   9   10   Stuffed
Foods/Amounts

Lunch   Time _____
Hunger/Fullness Scale:
Starving   1   2   3   4   5   6   7   8   9   10   Stuffed
Foods/Amounts

Dinner   Time _____
Hunger/Fullness Scale:
Starving   1   2   3   4   5   6   7   8   9   10   Stuffed
Foods/Amounts

🥨 *Snack*   Time _____

Hunger/Fullness Scale:

Starving   1   2   3   4   5   6   7   8   9   10   Stuffed

Foods/Amounts

Journal

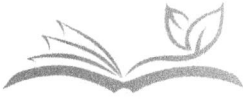

Was the food planned prior to starting the day?

❏ Yes   ❏ No

3 Credits

How many days have you followed a plan? _____

Did you follow your plan?

❏ Yes   ❏ No

If not, why? If yes – how did it feel?

Vitamins:

Multi • Probiotic • B Complex • Vitamin D
Calcium/Magnesium • Omega

Day ___: Make Today an Amen Day

Pleasant words are a honeycomb, sweet to the soul and healing to the bones.

Proverbs 16:24

Date _____   Water 1 2 3 4 5 6 7 8 9

Breakfast   Time _____
Hunger/Fullness Scale:

Starving   1   2   3   4   5   6   7   8   9   10   Stuffed

Foods/Amounts

Lunch   Time _____
Hunger/Fullness Scale:

Starving   1   2   3   4   5   6   7   8   9   10   Stuffed

Foods/Amounts

Dinner   Time _____
Hunger/Fullness Scale:

Starving   1   2   3   4   5   6   7   8   9   10   Stuffed

Foods/Amounts

🐦 *Snack*　　　　　Time _____

Hunger/Fullness Scale:

Starving　1　2　3　4　5　6　7　8　9　10　Stuffed

Foods/Amounts

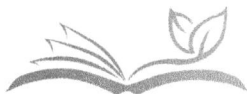

Was the food planned prior to starting the day?

❑ Yes　　❑ No

How many days have you followed a plan? _____

Did you follow your plan?

❑ Yes　　❑ No

If not, why? If yes – how did it feel?

Vitamins:

Multi • Probiotic • B Complex • Vitamin D
Calcium/Magnesium • Omega

3 Credits

My Advantage

Day ___: Make Today an Amen Day

*You shall love the Lord your God with all your heart and
with all your soul and with all your might.*

Deuteronomy 6:5

Date _____   Water 1 2 3 4 5 6 7 8 9

Breakfast   Time _____
Hunger/Fullness Scale:

Starving 1 2 3 4 5 6 7 8 9 10 Stuffed

Foods/Amounts

Lunch   Time _____
Hunger/Fullness Scale:

Starving 1 2 3 4 5 6 7 8 9 10 Stuffed

Foods/Amounts

Dinner   Time _____
Hunger/Fullness Scale:

Starving 1 2 3 4 5 6 7 8 9 10 Stuffed

Foods/Amounts

🏌 *Snack*   Time _____

Hunger/Fullness Scale:

Starving 1 2 3 4 5 6 7 8 9 10 Stuffed

Foods/Amounts

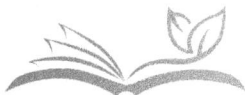

Was the food planned prior to starting the day?

❏ Yes   ❏ No

How many days have you followed a plan? _____

Did you follow your plan?

❏ Yes   ❏ No

If not, why? If yes – how did it feel?

Vitamins:

Multi • Probiotic • B Complex • Vitamin D
Calcium/Magnesium • Omega

Journal

3 Credits

Weekly Reflection

Take 5 to 10 minutes to reflect on your week. Always start from the perspective of what went well. Glance back at your credits. Focusing on the accomplishments directs the brain to continue in that pattern. The pattern of success.

Anticipate what the next seven days may include. Reflect on your eating, beliefs, and transformation tools; what needs more focus? Continue to offer up your prayers with thanksgiving!

God is at work and this journal is tracking His unique character in YOUR life.

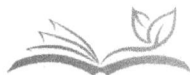

Prepare for the Next Week

As you review your personal calendar and see events or special gatherings, are there going to be any opportunities that may be a challenge?

Write that out now and decide how you are going to handle it.

Also make note of what days you are going to fast a meal. In the 40 Day Transformation Course it is taught for healthy living to fast 3 meals per week. These meals are totally your choice. Any day any meal.

Plan now your success in this area.

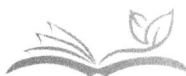

My Advantage

Day ___: Make Today an Amen Day

I discipline my body and make it my slave,
so that, after I have preached to others,
I myself will not be disqualified.

1 Corinthians 9:27

Date _____   Water 1 2 3 4 5 6 7 8 9

Breakfast   Time _____
Hunger/Fullness Scale:
Starving 1 2 3 4 5 6 7 8 9 10 Stuffed
Foods/Amounts

Lunch   Time _____
Hunger/Fullness Scale:
Starving 1 2 3 4 5 6 7 8 9 10 Stuffed
Foods/Amounts

Dinner   Time _____
Hunger/Fullness Scale:
Starving 1 2 3 4 5 6 7 8 9 10 Stuffed
Foods/Amounts

🫐 *Snack*   Time _____

Hunger/Fullness Scale:

Starving 1 2 3 4 5 6 7 8 9 10 Stuffed

Foods/Amounts

Journal

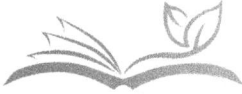

Was the food planned prior to starting the day?

❏ Yes   ❏ No

How many days have you followed a plan? _____

Did you follow your plan?

❏ Yes   ❏ No

If not, why? If yes – how did it feel?

Vitamins:

Multi • Probiotic • B Complex • Vitamin D
Calcium/Magnesium • Omega

3 Credits

Day ___: Make Today an Amen Day

*The steps of a man are established by the Lord,
and He delights in his way. When he falls, he
will not be hurled headlong, because the Lord
is the One who holds his hand.*

Psalms 37:23-24

Date _____   Water 1 2 3 4 5 6 7 8 9

Breakfast   Time _____
Hunger/Fullness Scale:
Starving 1 2 3 4 5 6 7 8 9 10 Stuffed
Foods/Amounts

Lunch   Time _____
Hunger/Fullness Scale:
Starving 1 2 3 4 5 6 7 8 9 10 Stuffed
Foods/Amounts

Dinner   Time _____
Hunger/Fullness Scale:
Starving 1 2 3 4 5 6 7 8 9 10 Stuffed
Foods/Amounts

🍩 *Snack* Time _____

Hunger/Fullness Scale:

Starving 1 2 3 4 5 6 7 8 9 10 Stuffed

Foods/Amounts

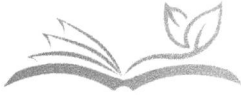

Was the food planned prior to starting the day?

❏ Yes   ❏ No

How many days have you followed a plan? _____

Did you follow your plan?

❏ Yes   ❏ No

If not, why? If yes – how did it feel?

Vitamins:

Multi • Probiotic • B Complex • Vitamin D
Calcium/Magnesium • Omega

3 Credits

Journal

My Advantage

Day ___: Make Today an Amen Day

He who is faithful in a very little thing is faithful also in much; and he who is unrighteous in a very little thing is unrighteous also in much. Therefore if you have not been faithful in the use of unrighteous wealth, who will entrust the true riches to you?

Luke 16:10-11

Date _____   Water 1 2 3 4 5 6 7 8 9

Breakfast   Time _____
Hunger/Fullness Scale:

Starving 1   2   3   4   5   6   7   8   9   10   Stuffed

Foods/Amounts

Lunch   Time _____
Hunger/Fullness Scale:

Starving 1   2   3   4   5   6   7   8   9   10   Stuffed

Foods/Amounts

Dinner   Time _____
Hunger/Fullness Scale:

Starving 1   2   3   4   5   6   7   8   9   10   Stuffed

Foods/Amounts

🍪 *Snack*　　　　Time _____

Hunger/Fullness Scale:

Starving　1　2　3　4　5　6　7　8　9　10　Stuffed

Foods/Amounts

Journal

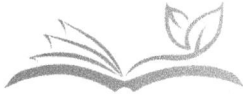

Was the food planned prior to starting the day?

❑ Yes　　❑ No

3 Credits

How many days have you followed a plan? _____

Did you follow your plan?

❑ Yes　　❑ No

If not, why? If yes – how did it feel?

Vitamins:

Multi • Probiotic • B Complex • Vitamin D

Calcium/Magnesium • Omega

Day ___: Make Today an Amen Day

So do not worry about tomorrow; for tomorrow will care
for itself. Each day has enough trouble of its own.

Matthew 6:34

Date _____   Water 1 2 3 4 5 6 7 8 9

Breakfast   Time _____
Hunger/Fullness Scale:

Starving   1   2   3   4   5   6   7   8   9   10   Stuffed

Foods/Amounts

Lunch   Time _____
Hunger/Fullness Scale:

Starving   1   2   3   4   5   6   7   8   9   10   Stuffed

Foods/Amounts

Dinner   Time _____
Hunger/Fullness Scale:

Starving   1   2   3   4   5   6   7   8   9   10   Stuffed

Foods/Amounts

🫛 *Snack*　　　　Time _____

Hunger/Fullness Scale:

Starving　1　2　3　4　5　6　7　8　9　10　Stuffed

Foods/Amounts

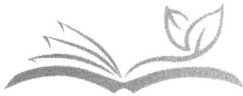

Was the food planned prior to starting the day?

❏ Yes　　❏ No

How many days have you followed a plan? _____

Did you follow your plan?

❏ Yes　　❏ No

If not, why? If yes – how did it feel?

Vitamins:

Multi • Probiotic • B Complex • Vitamin D
Calcium/Magnesium • Omega

Journal

3 Credits

My Advantage

Day ___: Make Today an Amen Day

If possible, so far as it depends on you,
be at peace with all men.

Romans 12:18

Date _____   Water 1 2 3 4 5 6 7 8 9

Breakfast   Time _____
Hunger/Fullness Scale:
Starving 1 2 3 4 5 6 7 8 9 10 Stuffed
Foods/Amounts

Lunch   Time _____
Hunger/Fullness Scale:
Starving 1 2 3 4 5 6 7 8 9 10 Stuffed
Foods/Amounts

Dinner   Time _____
Hunger/Fullness Scale:
Starving 1 2 3 4 5 6 7 8 9 10 Stuffed
Foods/Amounts

🍩 *Snack* Time _____

Hunger/Fullness Scale:

Starving 1 2 3 4 5 6 7 8 9 10 Stuffed

Foods/Amounts

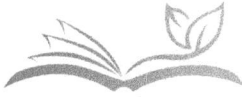

Was the food planned prior to starting the day?

❏ Yes   ❏ No

How many days have you followed a plan? _____

Did you follow your plan?

❏ Yes   ❏ No

If not, why? If yes – how did it feel?

Vitamins:

Multi • Probiotic • B Complex • Vitamin D
Calcium/Magnesium • Omega

Journal

3 Credits

Day ___: Make Today an Amen Day

*Rejoicing in hope, persevering in
tribulation, devoted to prayer.*

Romans 12:12

Date _____   Water 1 2 3 4 5 6 7 8 9

🌿 Breakfast   Time _____
Hunger/Fullness Scale:

Starving 1 2 3 4 5 6 7 8 9 10 Stuffed

Foods/Amounts

🌿 Lunch   Time _____
Hunger/Fullness Scale:

Starving 1 2 3 4 5 6 7 8 9 10 Stuffed

Foods/Amounts

🌿 Dinner   Time _____
Hunger/Fullness Scale:

Starving 1 2 3 4 5 6 7 8 9 10 Stuffed

Foods/Amounts

🍳 *Snack* Time _____

Hunger/Fullness Scale:

Starving 1 2 3 4 5 6 7 8 9 10 Stuffed

Foods/Amounts

Journal

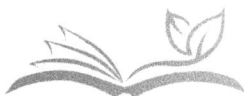

Was the food planned prior to starting the day?

❏ Yes   ❏ No

3 Credits

How many days have you followed a plan? _____

Did you follow your plan?

❏ Yes   ❏ No

If not, why? If yes – how did it feel?

Vitamins:

Multi • Probiotic • B Complex • Vitamin D
Calcium/Magnesium • Omega

Day ___: Make Today an Amen Day

Cast your burden upon the Lord and He will sustain you;
he will never allow the righteous to be shaken.

Psalm 55:22

Date _____   Water 1 2 3 4 5 6 7 8 9

Breakfast   Time _____
Hunger/Fullness Scale:
Starving 1 2 3 4 5 6 7 8 9 10 Stuffed
Foods/Amounts

Lunch   Time _____
Hunger/Fullness Scale:
Starving 1 2 3 4 5 6 7 8 9 10 Stuffed
Foods/Amounts

Dinner   Time _____
Hunger/Fullness Scale:
Starving 1 2 3 4 5 6 7 8 9 10 Stuffed
Foods/Amounts

🥨 *Snack*   Time _____

Hunger/Fullness Scale:

Starving 1 2 3 4 5 6 7 8 9 10 Stuffed

Foods/Amounts

Journal

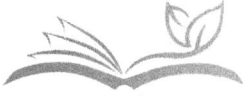

Was the food planned prior to starting the day?

❏ Yes   ❏ No

How many days have you followed a plan? _____

Did you follow your plan?

❏ Yes   ❏ No

If not, why? If yes – how did it feel?

Vitamins:

Multi • Probiotic • B Complex • Vitamin D
Calcium/Magnesium • Omega

3 Credits

Weekly Reflection

T ake 5 to 10 minutes to reflect on your week. Always start from the perspective of what went well. Glance back at your credits. Focusing on the accomplishments directs the brain to continue in that pattern. The pattern of success.

Anticipate what the next seven days may include. Reflect on your eating, beliefs, and transformation tools; what needs more focus? Continue to offer up your prayers with thanksgiving!

God is at work and this journal is tracking His unique character in YOUR life.

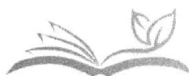

Prepare for the Next Week

As you review your personal calendar and see events or special gatherings, are there going to be any opportunities that may be a challenge?

Write that out now and decide how you are going to handle it.

Also make note of what days you are going to fast a meal. In the 40 Day Transformation Course it is taught for healthy living to fast 3 meals per week. These meals are totally your choice. Any day any meal.

Plan now your success in this area.

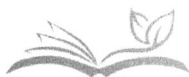

Journal

My Advantage

Day ___: Make Today an Amen Day

The mind of the prudent acquires knowledge,
and the ear of the wise seeks knowledge.

Proverbs 18:15

Date _____   Water 1 2 3 4 5 6 7 8 9

🫓 *Breakfast*   Time _____
Hunger/Fullness Scale:

Starving 1 2 3 4 5 6 7 8 9 10 Stuffed

Foods/Amounts

🫓 *Lunch*   Time _____
Hunger/Fullness Scale:

Starving 1 2 3 4 5 6 7 8 9 10 Stuffed

Foods/Amounts

🫓 *Dinner*   Time _____
Hunger/Fullness Scale:

Starving 1 2 3 4 5 6 7 8 9 10 Stuffed

Foods/Amounts

🍪 *Snack* Time _____

Hunger/Fullness Scale:

Starving 1 2 3 4 5 6 7 8 9 10 Stuffed

Foods/Amounts

Journal

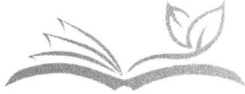

Was the food planned prior to starting the day?

❑ Yes   ❑ No

3 Credits

How many days have you followed a plan? _____

Did you follow your plan?

❑ Yes   ❑ No

If not, why? If yes – how did it feel?

Vitamins:

Multi • Probiotic • B Complex • Vitamin D
Calcium/Magnesium • Omega

Day ___: Make Today an Amen Day

And forgive us our debts, as we also
have forgiven our debtors.

Matthew 6:12

Date _____   Water 1 2 3 4 5 6 7 8 9

Breakfast   Time _____
Hunger/Fullness Scale:
Starving   1   2   3   4   5   6   7   8   9   10   Stuffed
Foods/Amounts

Lunch   Time _____
Hunger/Fullness Scale:
Starving   1   2   3   4   5   6   7   8   9   10   Stuffed
Foods/Amounts

Dinner   Time _____
Hunger/Fullness Scale:
Starving   1   2   3   4   5   6   7   8   9   10   Stuffed
Foods/Amounts

🍽 *Snack*　　　　　　Time _____

Hunger/Fullness Scale:

Starving　1　2　3　4　5　6　7　8　9　10　Stuffed

Foods/Amounts

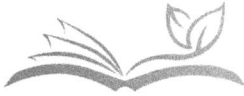

Was the food planned prior to starting the day?

❏ Yes　　❏ No

How many days have you followed a plan? _____

Did you follow your plan?

❏ Yes　　❏ No

If not, why? If yes – how did it feel?

Vitamins:

Multi • Probiotic • B Complex • Vitamin D
Calcium/Magnesium • Omega

Journal

3 Credits

Journal

My Advantage

Day ___: Make Today an Amen Day

But thanks be to God, who always leads us in triumph
in Christ, and manifests through us the sweet aroma
of the knowledge of Him in every place.

2 Corinthians 2:14

Date _____   Water 1 2 3 4 5 6 7 8 9

Breakfast   Time _____
Hunger/Fullness Scale:
Starving 1 2 3 4 5 6 7 8 9 10 Stuffed
Foods/Amounts

Lunch   Time _____
Hunger/Fullness Scale:
Starving 1 2 3 4 5 6 7 8 9 10 Stuffed
Foods/Amounts

Dinner   Time _____
Hunger/Fullness Scale:
Starving 1 2 3 4 5 6 7 8 9 10 Stuffed
Foods/Amounts

🥨 *Snack*   Time _____

Hunger/Fullness Scale:

Starving   1   2   3   4   5   6   7   8   9   10   Stuffed

Foods/Amounts

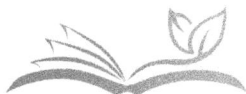

Was the food planned prior to starting the day?

❏ Yes   ❏ No

How many days have you followed a plan? _____

Did you follow your plan?

❏ Yes   ❏ No

If not, why? If yes – how did it feel?

Vitamins:

Multi • Probiotic • B Complex • Vitamin D
Calcium/Magnesium • Omega

Journal

3 Credits

Day ___: Make Today an Amen Day

And He said to them, "Come away by yourselves to a secluded place and rest a while."

Mark 6:31

Date _____   Water 1 2 3 4 5 6 7 8 9

🍃 *Breakfast*   Time _____
Hunger/Fullness Scale:

Starving 1 2 3 4 5 6 7 8 9 10 Stuffed

Foods/Amounts

🍃 *Lunch*   Time _____
Hunger/Fullness Scale:

Starving 1 2 3 4 5 6 7 8 9 10 Stuffed

Foods/Amounts

🍃 *Dinner*   Time _____
Hunger/Fullness Scale:

Starving 1 2 3 4 5 6 7 8 9 10 Stuffed

Foods/Amounts

🍪 *Snack*　　　　　Time _____

Hunger/Fullness Scale:

Starving　1　2　3　4　5　6　7　8　9　10　Stuffed

Foods/Amounts

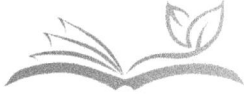

Was the food planned prior to starting the day?

❏ Yes　　❏ No

How many days have you followed a plan? _____

Did you follow your plan?

❏ Yes　　❏ No

If not, why? If yes – how did it feel?

Vitamins:

Multi • Probiotic • B Complex • Vitamin D
Calcium/Magnesium • Omega

Journal

3 Credits

My Advantage

Day ___: Make Today an Amen Day

Truly I say to you, whatever you bind on earth shall have been bound in heaven; and whatever you loose on earth shall have been loosed in heaven.

Matthew 18:18

Date _____   Water 1 2 3 4 5 6 7 8 9

Breakfast   Time _____
Hunger/Fullness Scale:

Starving 1 2 3 4 5 6 7 8 9 10 Stuffed

Foods/Amounts

Lunch   Time _____
Hunger/Fullness Scale:

Starving 1 2 3 4 5 6 7 8 9 10 Stuffed

Foods/Amounts

Dinner   Time _____
Hunger/Fullness Scale:

Starving 1 2 3 4 5 6 7 8 9 10 Stuffed

Foods/Amounts

✏️ *Snack*   Time _____

Journal

Hunger/Fullness Scale:

Starving 1 2 3 4 5 6 7 8 9 10 Stuffed

Foods/Amounts

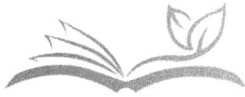

Was the food planned prior to starting the day?

❏ Yes   ❏ No

3 Credits

How many days have you followed a plan? _____

Did you follow your plan?

❏ Yes   ❏ No

If not, why? If yes – how did it feel?

Vitamins:

Multi • Probiotic • B Complex • Vitamin D
Calcium/Magnesium • Omega

Day ___: Make Today an Amen Day

*In peace I will both lie down and sleep, for
You alone, O Lord, make me to dwell in safety.*

Psalm4:8

Date _____   Water 1 2 3 4 5 6 7 8 9

🥗 *Breakfast*   Time _____
Hunger/Fullness Scale:

Starving 1   2   3   4   5   6   7   8   9   10   Stuffed

Foods/Amounts

🥗 *Lunch*   Time _____
Hunger/Fullness Scale:

Starving 1   2   3   4   5   6   7   8   9   10   Stuffed

Foods/Amounts

🥗 *Dinner*   Time _____
Hunger/Fullness Scale:

Starving 1   2   3   4   5   6   7   8   9   10   Stuffed

Foods/Amounts

🍪 *Snack*　　　　　Time _____

Hunger/Fullness Scale:

Starving　1　2　3　4　5　6　7　8　9　10　Stuffed

Foods/Amounts

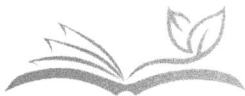

Was the food planned prior to starting the day?

❏ Yes　　❏ No

How many days have you followed a plan? _____

Did you follow your plan?

❏ Yes　　❏ No

If not, why? If yes – how did it feel?

Vitamins:

Multi • Probiotic • B Complex • Vitamin D
Calcium/Magnesium • Omega

Day ___: Make Today an Amen Day

When you lie down, you will not be afraid;
When you lie down, your sleep will be sweet.

Proverbs 3:24

Date _____   Water 1 2 3 4 5 6 7 8 9

Breakfast   Time _____
Hunger/Fullness Scale:
Starving 1 2 3 4 5 6 7 8 9 10 Stuffed
Foods/Amounts

Lunch   Time _____
Hunger/Fullness Scale:
Starving 1 2 3 4 5 6 7 8 9 10 Stuffed
Foods/Amounts

Dinner   Time _____
Hunger/Fullness Scale:
Starving 1 2 3 4 5 6 7 8 9 10 Stuffed
Foods/Amounts

🫓 *Snack*   Time _____

Hunger/Fullness Scale:

Starving   1   2   3   4   5   6   7   8   9   10   Stuffed

Foods/Amounts

Journal

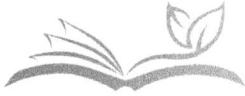

Was the food planned prior to starting the day?

❏ Yes   ❏ No

3 Credits

How many days have you followed a plan? _____

Did you follow your plan?

❏ Yes   ❏ No

If not, why? If yes – how did it feel?

Vitamins:

Multi • Probiotic • B Complex • Vitamin D
Calcium/Magnesium • Omega

Hunger ~ Satisfied Tastimony
Weekly Reflection

Take 5 to 10 minutes to reflect on your week. Always start from the perspective of what went well. Glance back at your credits. Focusing on the accomplishments directs the brain to continue in that pattern. The pattern of success.

Anticipate what the next seven days may include. Reflect on your eating, beliefs, and transformation tools; what needs more focus? Continue to offer up your prayers with thanksgiving!

God is at work and this journal is tracking His unique character in YOUR life.

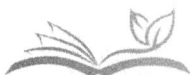

Prepare for the Next Week

As you review your personal calendar and see events or special gatherings, are there going to be any opportunities that may be a challenge?

Write that out now and decide how you are going to handle it.

Also make note of what days you are going to fast a meal. In the 40 Day Transformation Course it is taught for healthy living to fast 3 meals per week. These meals are totally your choice. Any day any meal.

Plan now your success in this area.

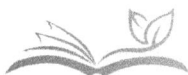

Day ___: Make Today an Amen Day

*We will stand before this house and before You
(for Your name is in this house) and cry to You in
our distress, and You will hear and deliver us.'*

2 Chronicles 20:9b

Date _____   Water 1 2 3 4 5 6 7 8 9

🥗 Breakfast   Time _____

Hunger/Fullness Scale:

Starving   1   2   3   4   5   6   7   8   9   10   Stuffed

Foods/Amounts

🥗 Lunch   Time _____

Hunger/Fullness Scale:

Starving   1   2   3   4   5   6   7   8   9   10   Stuffed

Foods/Amounts

🥗 Dinner   Time _____

Hunger/Fullness Scale:

Starving   1   2   3   4   5   6   7   8   9   10   Stuffed

Foods/Amounts

🍪 *Snack* Time _____

Hunger/Fullness Scale:

Starving 1 2 3 4 5 6 7 8 9 10 Stuffed

Foods/Amounts

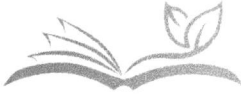

Was the food planned prior to starting the day?

❏ Yes   ❏ No

3 Credits

How many days have you followed a plan? _____

Did you follow your plan?

❏ Yes   ❏ No

If not, why? If yes – how did it feel?

Vitamins:

Multi • Probiotic • B Complex • Vitamin D
Calcium/Magnesium • Omega

My Advantage

Day ___: Make Today an Amen Day

He gives strength to the weary, and to him
who lacks might He increases power.

Isaiah 40:29

Date _____   Water 1 2 3 4 5 6 7 8 9

Breakfast   Time _____
Hunger/Fullness Scale:

Starving 1 2 3 4 5 6 7 8 9 10 Stuffed
Foods/Amounts

Lunch   Time _____
Hunger/Fullness Scale:

Starving 1 2 3 4 5 6 7 8 9 10 Stuffed
Foods/Amounts

Dinner   Time _____
Hunger/Fullness Scale:

Starving 1 2 3 4 5 6 7 8 9 10 Stuffed
Foods/Amounts

🎾 *Snack*　　　　Time _____

Hunger/Fullness Scale:

Starving 1 2 3 4 5 6 7 8 9 10 Stuffed

Foods/Amounts

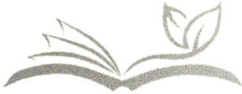

Was the food planned prior to starting the day?

❏ Yes　　❏ No

How many days have you followed a plan? _____

Did you follow your plan?

❏ Yes　　❏ No

If not, why? If yes – how did it feel?

Vitamins:

Multi • Probiotic • B Complex • Vitamin D
Calcium/Magnesium • Omega

Journal

3 Credits

Day ___: Make Today an Amen Day

*Yet those who wait for the Lord will gain new strength;
they will mount up with wings like eagles, they will run
and not get tired, they will walk and not become weary.*

Isaiah 40:31

Date _____   Water 1 2 3 4 5 6 7 8 9

Breakfast   Time _____
Hunger/Fullness Scale:
Starving 1   2   3   4   5   6   7   8   9   10   Stuffed
Foods/Amounts

Lunch   Time _____
Hunger/Fullness Scale:
Starving 1   2   3   4   5   6   7   8   9   10   Stuffed
Foods/Amounts

Dinner   Time _____
Hunger/Fullness Scale:
Starving 1   2   3   4   5   6   7   8   9   10   Stuffed
Foods/Amounts

🍪 *Snack*　　　　Time _____

Hunger/Fullness Scale:

Starving　1　2　3　4　5　6　7　8　9　10　Stuffed

Foods/Amounts

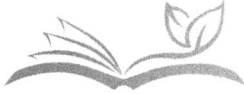

Was the food planned prior to starting the day?

❑ Yes　　❑ No

How many days have you followed a plan? _____

Did you follow your plan?

❑ Yes　　❑ No

If not, why? If yes – how did it feel?

Vitamins:

Multi • Probiotic • B Complex • Vitamin D
Calcium/Magnesium • Omega

Journal

3 Credits

My Advantage

Day ___: Make Today an Amen Day

For a sanctify Christ as Lord in your hearts, always being ready to make a defense to everyone who asks you to give an account for the hope that is in you.

1 Peter 3:15a

Date _____   Water 1 2 3 4 5 6 7 8 9

Breakfast   Time _____
Hunger/Fullness Scale:
Starving 1 2 3 4 5 6 7 8 9 10 Stuffed
Foods/Amounts

Lunch   Time _____
Hunger/Fullness Scale:
Starving 1 2 3 4 5 6 7 8 9 10 Stuffed
Foods/Amounts

Dinner   Time _____
Hunger/Fullness Scale:
Starving 1 2 3 4 5 6 7 8 9 10 Stuffed
Foods/Amounts

🍽 *Snack*   Time _____

Hunger/Fullness Scale:

Starving   1   2   3   4   5   6   7   8   9   10   Stuffed

Foods/Amounts

Journal

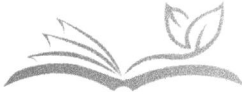

Was the food planned prior to starting the day?

❏ Yes   ❏ No

3 Credits

How many days have you followed a plan? _____

Did you follow your plan?

❏ Yes   ❏ No

If not, why? If yes – how did it feel?

Vitamins:

Multi • Probiotic • B Complex • Vitamin D
Calcium/Magnesium • Omega

My Advantage

Day ___: Make Today an Amen Day

Therefore I urge you, brethren, by the mercies of God, to present your bodies a living and holy sacrifice, acceptable to God, which is your spiritual service of worship.

Romans 12:1

Date _____   Water 1 2 3 4 5 6 7 8 9

🍳 *Breakfast*   Time _____
Hunger/Fullness Scale:

Starving 1 2 3 4 5 6 7 8 9 10 Stuffed

Foods/Amounts

🍽 *Lunch*   Time _____
Hunger/Fullness Scale:

Starving 1 2 3 4 5 6 7 8 9 10 Stuffed

Foods/Amounts

🍽 *Dinner*   Time _____
Hunger/Fullness Scale:

Starving 1 2 3 4 5 6 7 8 9 10 Stuffed

Foods/Amounts

🍪 *Snack*　　　　Time _____

Hunger/Fullness Scale:

Starving　1　2　3　4　5　6　7　8　9　10　Stuffed

Foods/Amounts

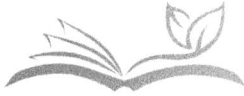

Was the food planned prior to starting the day?

❏ Yes　　❏ No

How many days have you followed a plan? _____

Did you follow your plan?

❏ Yes　　❏ No

If not, why? If yes – how did it feel?

Vitamins:

Multi • Probiotic • B Complex • Vitamin D
Calcium/Magnesium • Omega

Journal

My Advantage

Day ___: Make Today an Amen Day

And do not be conformed to this world, but be transformed by the renewing of your mind, so that you may prove what the will of God is, that which is good and acceptable and perfect.

Romans 12:2

Date _____   Water 1 2 3 4 5 6 7 8 9

Breakfast   Time _____
Hunger/Fullness Scale:
Starving 1 2 3 4 5 6 7 8 9 10 Stuffed
Foods/Amounts

Lunch   Time _____
Hunger/Fullness Scale:
Starving 1 2 3 4 5 6 7 8 9 10 Stuffed
Foods/Amounts

Dinner   Time _____
Hunger/Fullness Scale:
Starving 1 2 3 4 5 6 7 8 9 10 Stuffed
Foods/Amounts

🫐 *Snack*   Time _____

Hunger/Fullness Scale:

Starving   1   2   3   4   5   6   7   8   9   10   Stuffed

Foods/Amounts

Journal

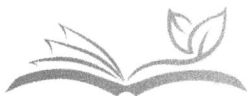

Was the food planned prior to starting the day?

❏ Yes   ❏ No

3 Credits

How many days have you followed a plan? _____

Did you follow your plan?

❏ Yes   ❏ No

If not, why? If yes – how did it feel?

Vitamins:

Multi • Probiotic • B Complex • Vitamin D
Calcium/Magnesium • Omega

Day ___: Make Today an Amen Day

Who is the one who is victorious and overcomes the world? It is the one who believes and recognizes the fact that Jesus is the Son of God.

1 John 5:5

Date _____   Water 1 2 3 4 5 6 7 8 9

Breakfast   Time _____
Hunger/Fullness Scale:

Starving 1 2 3 4 5 6 7 8 9 10 Stuffed

Foods/Amounts

Lunch   Time _____
Hunger/Fullness Scale:

Starving 1 2 3 4 5 6 7 8 9 10 Stuffed

Foods/Amounts

Dinner   Time _____
Hunger/Fullness Scale:

Starving 1 2 3 4 5 6 7 8 9 10 Stuffed

Foods/Amounts

🍋 *Snack*   Time _____

Hunger/Fullness Scale:

Starving 1 2 3 4 5 6 7 8 9 10 Stuffed

Foods/Amounts

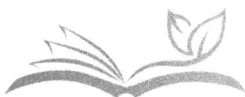

Was the food planned prior to starting the day?

❑ Yes   ❑ No

How many days have you followed a plan? _____

Did you follow your plan?

❑ Yes   ❑ No

If not, why? If yes – how did it feel?

Vitamins:

Multi • Probiotic • B Complex • Vitamin D
Calcium/Magnesium • Omega

Weekly Reflection

Take 5 to 10 minutes to reflect on your week. Always start from the perspective of what went well. Glance back at your credits. Focusing on the accomplishments directs the brain to continue in that pattern. The pattern of success.

Anticipate what the next seven days may include. Reflect on your eating, beliefs, and transformation tools; what needs more focus? Continue to offer up your prayers with thanksgiving!

God is at work and this journal is tracking His unique character in YOUR life.

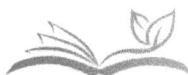

Prepare for the Next Week

As you review your personal calendar and see events or special gatherings, are there going to be any opportunities that may be a challenge?

Write that out now and decide how you are going to handle it.

Also make note of what days you are going to fast a meal. In the 40 Day Transformation Course it is taught for healthy living to fast 3 meals per week. These meals are totally your choice. Any day any meal.

Plan now your success in this area.

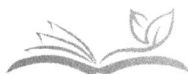

Day ___: Make Today an Amen Day

For the kingdom of God is not eating and drinking, but
righteousness and peace and joy in the Holy Spirit.
                                                Romans 14:17-18

Date _____   Water 1 2 3 4 5 6 7 8 9

Breakfast   Time _____
Hunger/Fullness Scale:
Starving 1 2 3 4 5 6 7 8 9 10 Stuffed
Foods/Amounts

Lunch   Time _____
Hunger/Fullness Scale:
Starving 1 2 3 4 5 6 7 8 9 10 Stuffed
Foods/Amounts

Dinner   Time _____
Hunger/Fullness Scale:
Starving 1 2 3 4 5 6 7 8 9 10 Stuffed
Foods/Amounts

🥨 *Snack*   Time _____

Hunger/Fullness Scale:

Starving 1 2 3 4 5 6 7 8 9 10 Stuffed

Foods/Amounts

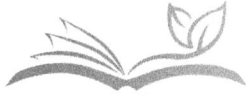

Was the food planned prior to starting the day?

❏ Yes   ❏ No

3 Credits

How many days have you followed a plan? _____

Did you follow your plan?

❏ Yes   ❏ No

If not, why? If yes – how did it feel?

Vitamins:

Multi • Probiotic • B Complex • Vitamin D
Calcium/Magnesium • Omega

Day ___: Make Today an Amen Day

Then he said to them, "Go, eat of the fat, drink of the sweet, and send portions to him who has nothing prepared; for this day is holy to our Lord. Do not be grieved, for the joy of the Lord is your strength.

Nehemiah 8:10

Date _____   Water 1 2 3 4 5 6 7 8 9

Breakfast   Time _____
Hunger/Fullness Scale:
Starving 1 2 3 4 5 6 7 8 9 10 Stuffed
Foods/Amounts

Lunch   Time _____
Hunger/Fullness Scale:
Starving 1 2 3 4 5 6 7 8 9 10 Stuffed
Foods/Amounts

Dinner   Time _____
Hunger/Fullness Scale:
Starving 1 2 3 4 5 6 7 8 9 10 Stuffed
Foods/Amounts

🫐 *Snack*   Time _____

Hunger/Fullness Scale:

Starving   1   2   3   4   5   6   7   8   9   10   Stuffed

Foods/Amounts

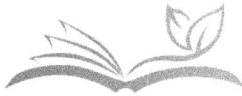

Was the food planned prior to starting the day?

❏ Yes   ❏ No

How many days have you followed a plan? _____

Did you follow your plan?

❏ Yes   ❏ No

If not, why? If yes – how did it feel?

Vitamins:

Multi • Probiotic • B Complex • Vitamin D
Calcium/Magnesium • Omega

Journal

3 Credits

Day ___: Make Today an Amen Day

Devote yourselves to prayer, keeping alert
in it with an attitude of thanksgiving.

Colossions 4:2

Date _____   Water 1 2 3 4 5 6 7 8 9

Breakfast   Time _____
Hunger/Fullness Scale:
Starving 1 2 3 4 5 6 7 8 9 10 Stuffed
Foods/Amounts

Lunch   Time _____
Hunger/Fullness Scale:
Starving 1 2 3 4 5 6 7 8 9 10 Stuffed
Foods/Amounts

Dinner   Time _____
Hunger/Fullness Scale:
Starving 1 2 3 4 5 6 7 8 9 10 Stuffed
Foods/Amounts

🥬 *Snack*   Time _____

Hunger/Fullness Scale:

Starving 1 2 3 4 5 6 7 8 9 10 Stuffed

Foods/Amounts

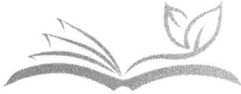

Was the food planned prior to starting the day?

❑ Yes   ❑ No

3 Credits

How many days have you followed a plan? _____

Did you follow your plan?

❑ Yes   ❑ No

If not, why? If yes – how did it feel?

Vitamins:

Multi • Probiotic • B Complex • Vitamin D
Calcium/Magnesium • Omega

My Advantage

Day ___: Make Today an Amen Day

Give thanks to the Lord, for He is good;
for His loving kindness is everlasting.

Psalm 118:1

Date _____   Water 1 2 3 4 5 6 7 8 9

🍃 *Breakfast*   Time _____
Hunger/Fullness Scale:
Starving 1   2   3   4   5   6   7   8   9   10   Stuffed
Foods/Amounts

🍃 *Lunch*   Time _____
Hunger/Fullness Scale:
Starving 1   2   3   4   5   6   7   8   9   10   Stuffed
Foods/Amounts

🍃 *Dinner*   Time _____
Hunger/Fullness Scale:
Starving 1   2   3   4   5   6   7   8   9   10   Stuffed
Foods/Amounts

🫐 *Snack*   Time _____

Hunger/Fullness Scale:

Starving 1 2 3 4 5 6 7 8 9 10 Stuffed

Foods/Amounts

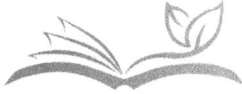

Was the food planned prior to starting the day?

❏ Yes   ❏ No

How many days have you followed a plan? _____

Did you follow your plan?

❏ Yes   ❏ No

If not, why? If yes – how did it feel?

Vitamins:

Multi • Probiotic • B Complex • Vitamin D

Calcium/Magnesium • Omega

Journal

3 Credits

Journal

My Advantage

Day ___: Make Today an Amen Day

*Whatever you do in word or deed, do all
in the name of the Lord Jesus, giving thanks
through Him to God the Father.*

Colossions 3:17

Date _____   Water 1 2 3 4 5 6 7 8 9

Breakfast   Time _____
Hunger/Fullness Scale:
Starving 1 2 3 4 5 6 7 8 9 10 Stuffed
Foods/Amounts

Lunch   Time _____
Hunger/Fullness Scale:
Starving 1 2 3 4 5 6 7 8 9 10 Stuffed
Foods/Amounts

Dinner   Time _____
Hunger/Fullness Scale:
Starving 1 2 3 4 5 6 7 8 9 10 Stuffed
Foods/Amounts

🍃 *Snack*　　　Time _____

Hunger/Fullness Scale:

Starving　1　2　3　4　5　6　7　8　9　10　Stuffed

Foods/Amounts

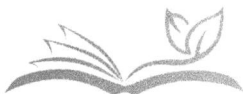

Was the food planned prior to starting the day?

❏ Yes　　❏ No

3 Credits

How many days have you followed a plan? _____

Did you follow your plan?

❏ Yes　　❏ No

If not, why? If yes – how did it feel?

Vitamins:

Multi • Probiotic • B Complex • Vitamin D
Calcium/Magnesium • Omega

Journal

My Advantage

Day ___: Make Today an Amen Day

But He answered and said, "It is written, 'Man shall not live on bread alone, but on every word that proceeds out of the mouth of God.'"

Matthew 4:4

Date _____   Water 1 2 3 4 5 6 7 8 9

Breakfast   Time _____
Hunger/Fullness Scale:
Starving   1   2   3   4   5   6   7   8   9   10   Stuffed
Foods/Amounts

Lunch   Time _____
Hunger/Fullness Scale:
Starving   1   2   3   4   5   6   7   8   9   10   Stuffed
Foods/Amounts

Dinner   Time _____
Hunger/Fullness Scale:
Starving   1   2   3   4   5   6   7   8   9   10   Stuffed
Foods/Amounts

🍩 *Snack*　　　Time _____

Hunger/Fullness Scale:

Starving　1　2　3　4　5　6　7　8　9　10　Stuffed

Foods/Amounts

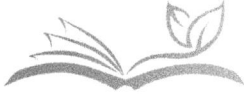

Was the food planned prior to starting the day?

❑ Yes　　❑ No

How many days have you followed a plan? _____

Did you follow your plan?

❑ Yes　　❑ No

If not, why? If yes – how did it feel?

Vitamins:

Multi • Probiotic • B Complex • Vitamin D
Calcium/Magnesium • Omega

Journal

3 Credits

My Advantage

Day ___: Make Today an Amen Day

Date _____   Water 1 2 3 4 5 6 7 8 9

Breakfast   Time _____
Hunger/Fullness Scale:

Starving 1 2 3 4 5 6 7 8 9 10 Stuffed

Foods/Amounts

Lunch   Time _____
Hunger/Fullness Scale:

Starving 1 2 3 4 5 6 7 8 9 10 Stuffed

Foods/Amounts

Dinner   Time _____
Hunger/Fullness Scale:

Starving 1 2 3 4 5 6 7 8 9 10 Stuffed

Foods/Amounts

🫐 *Snack*　　　　Time _____

Hunger/Fullness Scale:

Starving　1　2　3　4　5　6　7　8　9　10　Stuffed

Foods/Amounts

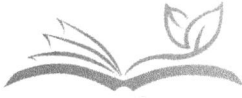

Was the food planned prior to starting the day?

❏ Yes　　❏ No

3 Credits

How many days have you followed a plan? _____

Did you follow your plan?

❏ Yes　　❏ No

If not, why? If yes – how did it feel?

Vitamins:

Multi • Probiotic • B Complex • Vitamin D
Calcium/Magnesium • Omega

Congratulations on completing this incredible life transforming journal.

This journal is beneficial for any area of life you desire greater rewards.

If you have not yet joined our membership coaching group then let me share what is happening there:

Biblical Nutrition Academy Coaching teaches you how to...

- ♣ Use your brain and God's Word to ease anxiety, stress, worry and boredom!
- ♣ Discover God's love for you on a whole new level!
- ♣ Process emotions and win!
- ♣ Motivate yourself physically and spiritually!
- ♣ Achieve your healthiest weight and health possible!
- ♣ See the person God created you to be and enjoy!
- ♣ Become confident in ALL areas of life!
- ♣ Experience breakthroughs!
- ♣ Truly KNOW how to pray for answers! No more doubting!
- ♣ Make meal time less stress with our Meal Prep coaching!

Biblical Nutrition Academy Coaching Membership is an all-inclusive monthly coaching program with training on these topics:

- ❧ Weight Loss
- ❧ Meal Prepping
- ❧ Praying the Answer
- ❧ Fasting
- ❧ Challenging Faulty Beliefs
- ❧ A Fresh Look at God's Words for YOU!
- ❧ PLUS MORE EACH MONTH!

Stay tuned to continue learning and enjoying God's recipe for excellent health

- ✓ Stay engaged on our blog: thebiblicalnutritionist.com/blog/

- ✓ Stay encouraged and entertained on our YouTube channel: The Biblical Nutritionist www.youtube.com/c/TheBiblicalNutritionist

- ✓ Stay excited with our recipes on our website: thebiblicalnutritionist.com/recipes

www.ingramcontent.com/pod-product-compliance
Lightning Source LLC
Chambersburg PA
CBHW031124020426
42333CB00012B/223